CHRONICLES OF BREAST CANCER SURVIVORS

Stories of Hope, Strength and Inspiration

Dr. ANAND KUMAR MISHRA

STARDOM BOOKS

www.StardomBooks.com

STARDOM BOOKS
A Division of Stardom Publishing
and infoYOGIS Technologies.
105-501 Silverside Road
Wilmington, DE 19809

FIRST EDITION JUNE 2022

STARDOM BOOKS

A Division of Stardom Alliance
105-501 Silverside Road Wilmington, DE 19809,
USA

www.stardombooks.com

Stardom Books, United States
Stardom Books, India
The author and publishers have made all reasonable
efforts to contact copyright-holders for permission,
and apologize for any omissions or errors in the
form of credits given. Corrections may be made to
future editions.

**CHRONICLES OF BREAST CANCER
SURVIVORS**
Stories of Hope, Strength and Inspiration

Dr. Anand Kumar Mishra

p. 232
cm. 13.5 X 21.5

Category:
MED058160 - Medical : Nursing - Oncology &
Cancer
HEA039030 - Health & Fitness : Diseases - Cancer

ISBN: 978-1-957456-08-9

DEDICATION

To my papa and late mummy [Shri S P Mishra, Vimala Mishra].

To all my patients and breast cancer survivors, for motivating me and making me realize the need to pen down my thoughts in the form of a book.

And, finally, my dear readers.
I sincerely hope you will understand the idea behind this book
— I would be the happiest if even a handful of you embraced the teachings mentioned in this book.

CONTENTS

ACKNOWLEDGMENTS

First, I bow down to the lotus feet of Guru Ji for his benediction. I appreciate Anjana, my wife, for standing by me, no matter what, and supporting me through all my endeavors.

My son and daughter (Aditya and Gauri) are precious gems who always stimulated and teased me while I was writing this book. I want to take this opportunity to thank AP Mishra and Arun Mishra (my elder brothers), Aparna (my sister), Bhavana and Aabha (my bhabhis), Dr. AB Singh, Abhay Singh, Dhru Singh, friends, colleagues in the 'Lucknow Breast Cancer Support Group,' and many others who motivated me to write this book.

This book would not have been possible without the dedicated support of all my patients and survivors. Many thanks to all my patients, who have knowingly and unknowingly pushed me to embark on this journey. I am grateful to all of you. Their personal stories have taught me about gratitude, compassion, listening, and acceptance.
I have stayed in touch with my patients, survivors, and their families, and they have taught me many "personal" lessons. I have seen many of the survivors totally transforming from introverted, shy individuals to the most helpful people and devoting every day of their lives toward helping others overcome their pain.

I owe a deep debt to God and bow before him for bestowing on me the creative imagination to write a book on the FEELINGS, FIGHT, and DETERMINATION of breast cancer survivors for the purpose of bringing HOPE. I avowedly feel the benevolence of Almighty God incessantly, and I pray to him to continue his blessings as well.

I would like to thank the team at Stardom Books for helping me through the editorial process and bringing out this book. Lastly, I value and respect each and every person who has been a part of this book. If I have unknowingly missed mentioning anyone's name, please know that your contribution is highly valued.

INTRODUCTION

The human body is made up of trillions of cells. A group of cells with similar structures and functions work together as a unit to form a tissue. An organ is a collection of tissues that form a functional unit and are specialized to perform a particular function. The human body has many major organ systems. Cancer is a disease in which the cells of an organ start growing uncontrollably and have the potential to spread to other parts of the body. The breast is an organ whose primary biological function is to produce milk to feed a baby. It is a symbol of femininity and beauty. Women's breasts are made of specialized tissues that produce milk (glandular tissue), fatty tissue, and a system of ducts that transport milk to the nipple. The milk-producing part of the breast is organized into 15 to 20 sections called lobes.

Its development is under the control of female hormones released by the ovaries at puberty. These hormones cause fat accumulation and enlargement of the breast. Breasts in men are rudimentary and do not develop in the absence of female hormones. The development of the breast starts in adolescence, and during pregnancy, the glandular component increases. The appearance of the normal female breast differs greatly from one woman to another.

The appearance can also vary at different times in a woman's life—before, during, and after adolescence, during pregnancy, during the menstrual cycle, and after menopause. Humans are the only life forms with permanent breasts. Every other mammal develops temporary breasts during ovulation or nursing in order to produce milk for their young.

Cancer can affect the breast gland too. It can start initially in the cells of either the glandular or the ductular system in the breast and later involve both these systems. Breast cancer is at present the single-most common cancer of women worldwide and the most likely reason for a woman to die of cancer. It is seen in all the countries irrespective of their economic status. And most of the deaths related to breast cancer occur in developing and under-developed nations. In fact, in developing nations, the maximum deaths occur due to the following three conditions: trauma, cancer, and communicable diseases. Cancer is a non-communicable disease, but it differs from other non-communicable diseases because it can be treated if detected early. In contrast, other non-communicable illnesses, such as diabetes and hypertension, require life-long treatment.

The diagnosis of any illness can be quite frightening, and it is more so when the diagnosis is cancer. The very words strike fear in a person's heart. And after the terrifying truth is confirmed, the world you live in is rocked badly. All of a sudden, there are so many details to take care of. You not only have to plan your treatment, but you also have to plan for the future. Arrangements to look after the family, especially the spouse and children, need to be made. All this has to be dealt with in the midst of your own fears and the well-meant condolences of friends and relatives. No wonder, then, many people diagnosed with the condition prefer to keep the matter within the close family circle. Dealing with curiosity and unasked-for advice can be daunting and draining.

All these are magnified when it is a woman. The life of a woman revolves around her family, and she is quick to identify anything that threatens the very fabric of the family. Hence, she will do anything, bear anything to keep the family's integrity. Their comfort and well-being are of paramount importance.

In India, women who hail from traditional family setups are conditioned to believe that the family comes first. This actually translates to husband, children, in-laws, and sundry other male members of the family. There is an inborn hesitancy to mention their illnesses and there could be many reasons for this. For one, they have always been seeing from childhood their own mothers and grandmothers in the nurturing role: always caring for the men and children in the family and making light of their own ailments. This leads her to believe it is just not done to fall sick and become a burden to the family, especially if she is married and living with her in-laws.

Breast cancer is a non-preventable cancer as its exact cause is unknown. However, women at a high risk of developing breast cancer can be identified based on the defined risk factors. This has been discussed in detail in further chapters of this book. Screening for breast cancer helps in its early detection, and most Western countries have well-organized screening programs in place. However, healthcare policymakers have been debating the strengths and limitations of mammography in breast cancer screening. In places where national screening programs are not in place, opportunistic screening must be undertaken for women in the high-risk group. Opportunistic screening involves screening for breast cancer when women visit a healthcare facility for any problem.

Breast cancer is seen on all the continents and affects females of all the countries with varied penetrance. Each region of the world and country has specific issues related to this cancer. Developing nations differ from developed nations in terms of stage of presentation.

Our country, India, has its own issues related to breast cancer. India is a subcontinent with wide ethnic, cultural, religious, and economic diversity and variation in the healthcare infrastructure. The healthcare facility pattern is heterogeneous, with numerous regions where the benefits of the awareness, early diagnosis, and multidisciplinary treatment programs have not reached. There are some unique issues in Indian breast cancer patients.

There is ignorance in the Indian society regarding this cancer and numerous myths associated with it as well. Women often do not present for medical care early enough due to various reasons, such as illiteracy, lack of awareness, and financial constraints. Women in developing countries, including India, are most often diagnosed with locally advanced (Stage 3) or metastatic (Stage 4) cancer. In later chapters, we have also explained about advanced breast cancer. Cancers in advanced stages are more expensive to treat and are less likely to respond to therapy. Indian patients are usually younger at presentation, with a greater proportion having aggressive forms of cancer. As most patients pay for their treatment, there is less affordability for targeted drugs. The quality of care available for breast cancer patients varies widely according to where the patient is being treated. There are centers of excellence providing multimodality protocol-based treatment at par with the best anywhere in the world, but these are few and located in big cities. It has been established beyond doubt that early diagnosis not only improves breast cancer outcomes but also makes the management less complicated and less expensive. Therefore, the need of the hour in low- and middle-income countries is to enable the early diagnosis of breast cancer at less advanced stages and decrease the delay in diagnosis or treatment initiation. Delay in diagnosis or treatment initiation is a modifiable determinant of outcomes. Delays can be classified as (1) patient delay, the period between the onset of symptoms and first medical consultation; and (2) system delay, time from the first consultation to treatment initiation.

There can be a delay in definitive diagnosis, or 'diagnosis delay,' and 'treatment delay' after the patient presents for the first consultation. Patient delay of longer than three months is a risk factor for the advanced stage at diagnosis. For metastatic disease, a treatment delay of 12 weeks or more is associated with worse survival. In non-metastatic disease, the negative impact of greater than 12 weeks treatment delay is seen in a more advanced stage of cancer at the time of treatment initiation.

In most developing nations, including India, healthcare facilities are heterogeneous in distribution; some cities have the best facilities while other areas have suboptimal facilities. These are reasons for 'system delay.' Policy makers need to prioritize the spending on breast cancer diagnosis and treatment by increasing cost-effective investments in prevention, early diagnosis, and access to care as these will shorten the 'patient delay.'

The median invasive tumor size at initial diagnosis and the ratio of advanced-stage to early-stage disease at initial diagnosis are two simple and powerful indicators of the efficacy of breast cancer detection programs in a particular country. These values indicate how good the early detection strategies of a country are. When the median invasive tumor size is between three to four centimeters, that region is said to have a lot of clinically detectable cancers. These regions will benefit from improving public knowledge about breast cancer and providing better healthcare facilities. Practical interventions to increase awareness include public education about the signs and symptoms of breast cancer, the advantages of early detection, and breast self-examination. The timely diagnosis of clinically detectable disease also requires facilities for diagnostic tissue sample analysis.

Ignorance of the symptoms of breast cancer and its treatment is a major issue for the delay in seeking treatment. In the case of breast cancer, the earliest symptom in many instances is a breast lump. This can be picked up by women in the early stages by performing regular breast self-examination. But for this, it is important that they first know about the disease, and then they also need to know about self-examination. The single most visible feature that defines a woman's appearance and femininity is thought to be the presence of shapely breasts. Of course, as a woman grows older, there are inevitable changes that occur, and the breasts lose their shape and firmness. And there are changes that take place in the breasts during the menstrual cycle as well.

Changes in the fluid content and the tissues can result in a feeling of heaviness and pain in many women during their menstrual cycle. These are normal cyclical symptoms that disappear after the periods and do not indicate cancer.

Because the breast is an important indicator of femininity and the most visible symbol that defines a woman, any disease that leads to the surgical excision of a breast can have devastating psychological effects on a woman. Owing to these reasons, surgery on the breasts should not be undertaken lightly. It is vital that surgeons keep the dual goals of cure and aesthetics in mind while operating. There have been instances where surgery on the breasts for benign conditions has resulted in ugly scarring or unwarranted changes in the size and shape of the breasts. Therefore, women must choose their breast surgeon very carefully.

The size and shape of the breasts are unique to every female. There is no consensus on the normal size of a breast or objective guidelines to describe the ideal shape of a breast. We often say that beauty lies in the eyes of the beholder. That is quite true! The perception of beauty varies greatly among patients and surgeons, and factors such as age, sex, and sociocultural background have a role to play in this. There are some defined measurements, which are universally accepted and used by breast surgeons to achieve the desired aesthetic results during breast surgery. The ideal breast shape is defined by the ratio of 45:55—45 percent of breast fullness above the nipple and 55 percent below the nipple.

Usually, the breasts on both sides are identical in size, shape, and firmness. However, a minor difference in size is acceptable, and up to 20 percent difference in volume between the right and left breast is considered normal. The nipple is situated seven to eight centimeters above the breast fold; the breast fold is where the breast meets the chest wall horizontally. The nipple is situated in the middle of the breast gland in the vertical plane and slightly lateral to the midpoint in the horizontal plane. The areola is generally 40 mm or lesser in diameter.

Ideally, the two nipples should form an equilateral triangle with the sternal notch. That is, the distance between the two nipples and the distance from a nipple to the sternal notch should measure the same, and it is normally between 19 cm and 21 cm.

The ideal cup size is said to be size C. For a pleasing and aesthetic appearance, the areolar diameter to the breast base width ratio and the nipple diameter to the areolar diameter should be 0.29. This is known as the "Rule of Thirds," which means that the areola represents just under one-third of the breast base width and the nipple represents approximately one-third of the areolar diameter. The height of the breast is usually more than two times of projection from the chest wall and the height to width of breast ratio is between 0.7 to 1. I have described these measurements just to give everybody an idea about the aesthetics of the breast. The size and shape of the breast are unique for every woman and depend on her body habitus. Often, young women use unproven creams and lotions to enhance their breast beauty. There is no proof that specialized food or diet plans, supplements, pumps, creams, or lotions can increase breast size or its beauty.

Breast cancer surgery involves two options: mastectomy and breast conservation surgery. Breast conservation surgery is usually the option in early-stage breast cancers or when the size of the tumor has decreased post-chemotherapy in advanced cancer. Excision of more than 20 percent of the breast tissue volume results in cosmetically unacceptable outcomes.

Today's patients are very concerned about the post-operative outcome and less accepting of poor aesthetic outcomes. Oncoplastic breast surgery is a technique by which volume is displaced in the defect area or replaced from non-breast areas. Volume displacement is a breast reshaping procedure where the principles of plastic surgery are applied and the site of the defect is filled with breast tissue from another portion of the breast. In volume replacement procedures, autologous tissues are used to replace the volume loss following tumor resection.

The adequacy of surgical management of breast cancer is always correlated with locoregional recurrence, which in turn correlates to the risk of death. One has to understand that adequate surgical management of breast cancer is fundamental to improving the outcomes irrespective of where cancer care is delivered. This is why I say that patients must choose their breast cancer surgeon carefully, as the first surgery is very important in terms of the outcome of disease as well as cosmesis. It is preferable that your surgeon is a specialist and not a jack-of-all-trades.

Cancer is generally considered a death warrant in our society, but it is not true. Timely and adequate treatment can provide a complete cure. Another very important factor that determines 'cure' is the pathology of cancer. **The Biology of the Cancer is the 'KING.'** It dictates the course of the disease, treatment outcomes, and long-term outcomes in a breast cancer patient. Biology, or in medical terms, histopathology can only be assessed after the biopsy of the mass. If tumor biology is bad, the patient will have a rapid downhill course and may not survive long, irrespective of the place of treatment.

A strong myth that I have been hearing consistently is the 'concern for biopsy.' Many of the patients do not want to have a biopsy and their attendants too agree with this. Their argument is that cancer cells spread faster after coming in contact with metal.

Now, not undergoing a biopsy does not help, and it unnecessarily delays the diagnosis and treatment. I want to assure all the breast cancer patients that biopsy does not cause any harm to you and it provides us with information about the biology of the tumor by which we plan the treatment. Breast cancer is curable in the early stages of the disease. However, patients with advanced or metastatic breast tumors have a lower chance of complete cure. Often, the aim of therapy in these patients is the control of disease by chemotherapy, which aims to stop the growth and spread of cancer and minimize the symptoms. Palliative care is where oncologists help cancer patients by treating the various symptoms of cancer spread.

End-of-life care is provided when nothing more can be done for the patient. Very often, women have doubts and queries regarding breast health. Breast cancer patients come across many myths associated with the disease. Lacking an authentic source for clearing their doubts, they look for answers from the people around them or resort to searching on the Internet.

"IDIOT syndrome" or 'Internet Derived Information Obstructing Treatment' is also a big problem in the present time and causes all types of delays (patient, diagnosis, and treatment). Patients should be knowledgeable about the disease and treatment. In fact, it is the sole purpose of all breast cancer awareness programs. For awareness campaigns, social media and the Internet are widely used, but as patients, you should be very careful when choosing the site for your information and knowledge. We often find people who are unrelated to the medical field blithely providing advice on hospitals, doctors, investigations, chemotherapy, and surgery. Some of these 'experts' would probably have never been acquainted with a breast cancer patient. When a patient suffers a recurrence of breast cancer, everyone considers it as the natural progression of the disease and they never attribute it to second-grade, ill-planned, ill-managed, and sub-optimal treatment. Only rarely do patients accept that they are at fault for choosing the wrong doctor, hospital, or treatment method. During my carrier spanning more than 25 years, I have come across many varieties of patients, and if I were to classify them, they often fall into one of the following seven categories:

1. **The patient who wants the doctor to make all the decisions or 'The Passive Dependent'**: These patients prefer to leave all aspects of healthcare decisions in the hands of their medical professional. They honestly feel that their doctor knows best. They have little or no interest in comprehending or discussing treatment risks and benefits.

2. **Open-Minded:** They have an honest relationship with the doctor. They want to thoroughly understand their problem and the treatment options and then come to a decision.

3. **The patient wants to act as the doctor in his or her way or 'The Independent Skeptic'**: These patients are the toughest to deal with. They are more likely to seek a second, third, or even fourth opinion and lose precious time in the process. There is always treatment delay leading to disease progression.

4. **The patient who does not want to consider surgery as an option or 'The Self-Destructive Denier'**: These patients do not want to undergo surgery. They drop out from treatment when surgery is advised and later come back with progression of the disease.

5. **The Researcher**: They will take the time to look up the best doctors from social media and the Internet and learn the latest treatments. They will read frequently about the treatment and will question the action of each drug and its use many times. They might sometimes choose the treatment depending upon their knowledge and not follow medical advice.

6. **The patient who just wants to verify the advice of another doctor or who comes for a second opinion or 'Explorer.'**

7. **The Patient is interested to switch practices or try other 'pathies.'**

Good patient characteristics include obedience, patience, politeness, listening, enthusiasm for treatment, intelligence, physical cleanliness, honesty, gratitude, and lifestyle adaptations. It is easy to deal with patients in category 1. They are basically obedient, patient, and polite. It takes effective communication skills to deal with patients in categories 2 and 3. The aim must be to convert patients in categories 4 to 7 into the first three categories using effective communication techniques to avoid treatment delays.

There are numerous instances where I have been the first contact person for patients. I have seen them, guided them through the various investigations, and confirmed the diagnosis of cancer. After the confirmation, they choose to leave and get treated with alternative remedies. This leads to cancer progression and treatment delay with dismal outcomes, ultimately.

Sometimes patients leave because I do not go by their wishes in the order of treatment. For instance, some patients want surgery immediately in the case of non-operable tumors instead of chemotherapy, which would have reduced tumor mass and allowed a better result in the following surgery. Many patients tend to consult multiple specialists. Getting a second opinion or even a third opinion is not wrong, but none of these consultations or 'opinions' are going to be of any benefit unless the treatment is started. Patients who go 'doctor shopping' should be discouraged as they usually do not follow anybody's advice. It only results in a waste of time, and meanwhile, cancer steadily progresses.

I have been affected emotionally many times by seeing the suffering of my patients. I would like to recount the instance of a patient with ulcerative breast cancer. She was a widow with two children and was working in a community kitchen for a paltry salary of Rs 800 per month. She approached me for a prescription form. I asked why she did not want to get treated for the disease. She answered that she could not afford to be absent from work as she would lose her job; she wanted the prescription slip to just show her children and convince them that she was indeed taking treatment. Patients have numerous reasons for not being able to undergo treatment. Every time I see a patient with advanced cancer, I feel very sorry and ask them why they came in so late. Each time there is a different answer. A few months back, a 70-year-old lady from a well-to-do family presented with advanced ulcerative breast cancer. The family members had become aware of her disease only the previous day and had rushed her to the hospital. When I talked to her, she told me that she had known about her condition for the past year, but had not disclosed it to her family members as she had been afraid that she would be isolated.

This book has sections on different aspects of breast cancer that people are not aware of and stories of many breast cancer survivors who underwent treatment at my department. The aim is to inform and educate everybody that breast cancer is indeed curable if diagnosed and treated early.

You will find this is the dominant theme of the book.

In the course of my professional career at the King George's Memorial University, Lucknow, I have been greatly influenced by the courage and determination shown by the many women with breast cancer whom I have treated. God has been very kind in providing me with an opportunity to treat patients from various backgrounds (residence, profession, education, affordability), with variable family composition (nuclear, single-parent, combined, or grandparent), from differing cultures, and of varied ethnicity, presenting at various stages of the disease. But all of them had a common suffering. I have seen one thing common in all of them: the 'determination to conquer the disease and be victorious.' Their confessions moved me a lot and stimulated me to draft a book so that everybody can benefit from their courage, determination, and confidence. There are many issues of survivorship after completion of treatment when the patient has achieved a cure. These include physical, mental, emotional, social, and sexual issues. A dedicated chapter has been included to highlight these issues.

In these deeply personal stories, these women have been unflinchingly honest as they recount the most difficult times in their lives, telling us how they found the strength and determination that they never knew they possessed.

Each one of them is a hero or heroine in my eyes, and each of their confessions has a unique perspective, which can be a source of inspiration and encouragement for newly diagnosed breast cancer patients. Each of these confessions invokes strength, hope, and confidence. The different chapters of the book have been designed around the stories of survivors to better understand the various issues of breast cancer. I hope this book will also be very useful in increasing the awareness of breast cancer. This book also addresses the numerous myths and taboos associated with breast cancer and provides insight and understanding of the general aspects of breast cancer treatment. I also believe this book will help break many of the barriers and help women speak out about their problems and health matters.

1

BREAST CANCER: NOT A TABOO

Talking about cancer helps remove the associated stigma and fear

Breast Cancer is the most common cancer prevalent among women across the world. It accounts for a third of all the cancers that affect women in the US. In recent years, breast cancer has preceded cervical cancer in terms of incidence as well as mortality. Once it was thought to affect only women from developed countries; however, breast cancer has now become a major health burden in developing countries. Indian breast cancer patients have an earlier age of onset (by 10 years) compared to the West. Moreover, the predominance of social taboos, absence of national breast cancer screening programs, and lack of awareness of the disease lead to the late diagnosis. Every four minutes, one Indian woman is diagnosed with cancer.

One in twenty-eight Indian women is likely to develop breast cancer during her lifetime. This ratio is higher (1 in 22) among urban women than that in rural women (1 in 60). About 80 percent of women diagnosed with breast cancer each year are aged 45 years or older, and about 43 percent are 65 years or older. In women aged 40 to 50 years, there is a 1 in 69 risk of developing breast cancer. From ages 50 to 60, the risk increases to 1 in 43. In the 60 to 70 age group, the risk is 1 in 29.

Cancer has been long associated with the stigma of being an incurable illness that leads to a lingering and painful death. This is a totally false perception. Cancer is potentially curable. We need to talk about cancer. And we need to talk about breast cancer! Frankly, Indian society nourishes a squeamish attitude toward womanhood and a women's body, and the prevailing patriarchal mentality often kindles a sense of fear and shame in women, leading to ignorance and an unforthcoming attitude.

In India, a girl is brought up to be gentle and filled with humility; a woman is bestowed with the endless responsibility of taking care of her family. A woman must be rational enough to put everyone's desires before her personal needs. Irrespective of her educational status or earning capacity, a woman's strength and femininity are thought to reside in her physical beauty and in her ability to give birth. But what if she falls sick or falls prey to a dreadful disease like Breast Cancer? Diagnosis of breast cancer can be the most frightening experience for any woman. The discovery of a lump in the breast, the impending fear of losing her breasts and beauty, and the social stigma associated with the disease make this the most harrowing phase of her life.

There prevails a feeling of uncertainty about the future and the treatment. Breast cancer is usually associated with a strong emotional component. Fear, societal misinformation, and the taboo associated with losing one's breasts often prevent a woman from seeking the treatment she needs. The stigma associated with Breast Cancer is unwarranted and BOGUS.

Breast Cancer is a completely curable disease and the survivors can lead a healthy and normal life after completing their treatment.

So why is there a fear of cancer among people?

Joseph Goebbels said, "A lie told a thousand times becomes the truth." A lie repeated a million times is often perceived as a fact. We as humans live out our lives with some preconceived notions.

Family heritage, religious beliefs, cultural background, educational qualifications, and societal ambiance play a role in shaping our views. Breast cancer is associated with an organ of femininity, sexuality, and motherhood, and the associated stigma is illustrated through exclusion, rejection, blame, or devaluation.

.

> "I do not feel any less of a woman. I feel empowered that I made a strong choice that no way diminishes my femininity.
> Angelina Jolie
> (On her double mastectomy)

Misconceptions and rumors spread faster than wildfire. The disgrace associated with the disease is so strong that patients are often blamed by their families for somehow bringing it on themselves. This should be condemned.

Many women fear abandonment by the community and hesitate to come forward for a proper diagnosis. Breast cancer is a disease that can affect the self-esteem of women and can take a toll on their relationships with their husbands and other family members. Societal prejudices call out a breast cancer patient as a sinner in God's eyes.

The humiliation associated with the diagnosis as well as the constant pressure to preserve one's womanly beauty often leads to intense emotional turmoil. Bringing the facts about Breast Cancer to light is essential to demystifying cancer. Women must be encouraged to look for signs of cancer, have regular mammograms, and seek professional support for breast symptoms.

There is also a strong need for campaigns teaching husbands and family members how to support the women in the house.

Let me share with you a proven statistical report. The Indian Women's Health Report 2021, surveying 1,000 working women aged between 25 and 55 across seven cities, has revealed that about half of the women surveyed were not comfortable talking about one or more women's health issues due to the prevalent societal taboo and stigma associated with them. The taboo around breast cancer is conceived in two forms—perceived and actual. The perceived stigma refers to the shame associated with having the disease and the fear of being discriminated against and denied basic respect and rights leading to social exclusion.

On the other hand, the actual stigma is about overt discrimination, which may lead to feelings of guilt and shame, and threaten one's own identity. It threatens the psychological and social aspects of life. The stigma associated with the disease is further compounded when the patient is held responsible for the condition and if the disease leads to severe disabilities, disfigurement, or any disruption of social interactions.

Losing hair following chemotherapy and losing a breast during surgery often generate anxiety and fear. There are fears and myths of incurability, pain, suffering, loss of control and independence, helplessness, isolation, loss of wages, poverty, and death. Many a time, family members can be a source of hindrance, particularly in rural areas. If the cancer patient belongs to the elderly age group, she may be deprived of care when she needs it the most. Furthermore, there is a social perception that a person having cancer is too ill to be employed, which makes the person's life difficult by curtailing employment opportunities. Thus, it becomes difficult for individuals with cancer to return to work or to try to secure new employment. Therefore, breast cancer is often kept a secret in the workplace. Women are extremely reluctant to disclose their symptoms related to breast or cervical cancer or any cancer involving the genital organs.

The willingness to undergo a general examination is low. Inherently, a woman is shy to talk about her private parts and is often reluctant to visit a male doctor. Many patients feel the diagnosis brings in the awful label of being a cancer patient. The labeling comes in various forms: through the appearance of perceived signs or symptoms of cancer or treatment side effects or cancer diagnosis by a health professional. Furthermore, a lot of misconceptions and myths regarding magical cures or remedies by quacks/faith healers delay care-seeking behavior. This is also one of the factors for delay in presentation, diagnosis, and initiation of proper treatment. Patient-physician communication remains an essential and critical step for mitigating the stigma associated with breast cancer. The diagnosis of cancer is many a time concealed from the patient due to the insistence of families, sociocultural norms, and the burden it brings alongside it. This obviously affects further decision-making and the development of coping strategies in the case of the patient.

The patient-doctor relationship is one of mutual trust, and all information regarding the patient's health should be discussed, and the treatment plan should be finalized only after extensive discussion with important family members and the primary caregiver. Public education and awareness campaigns can be reinforcing factors for building health literacy about breast cancer stigma. Awareness campaigns in schools and colleges can be of great help in changing societal perceptions. The stories of cancer survivors who successfully beat the disease can be of great help in reducing fear and invoking hope and confidence.

Here are two fascinating stories of my survivors, which I wish to share. Anju received treatment for right-sided breast carcinoma in 2014–2015 and is now cured completely. However, she has developed lymphedema in the right arm. Anita was diagnosed with triple-negative left breast cancer, and she received chemotherapy followed by surgery and radiation.

Both are very active members of our 'Lucknow Breast Cancer Support Group' and are always ready to help other patients.

SURVIVOR NOTES

Name: Anju Verma
Age- 54 years
Place- Lucknow

I am Anju Verma, a 54-year-old resident of Lucknow. I am also a proud breast cancer survivor. That is my identity now. I am not sure where to start my story; however, I am sharing my experience in the belief that it can bring a difference in how women take care of themselves. I hope my battle with breast cancer shall be an inspiration to many. In 2014, my husband was felicitated at his workplace for 25 years of meritorious service. While getting ready for the function, I noticed a slight retraction in my right nipple. I looked carefully in the mirror, and yes, there was a slight change. Two years earlier, I had undergone surgery for the removal of two breast lumps. At that time, the doctors had told me not to worry as the lumps were benign. We consulted the doctor the very next day. When he saw the nipple retraction, the doctor suspected a probable malignancy and prescribed a series of tests, such as FNAC, ultrasound scanning, and mammography.

The reports of all the tests came back negative for cancer. The doctor referred me to a consultant surgeon who was experienced in breast cancer management. Notwithstanding the negative test results, the surgeon felt it was best to operate based on my history of breast lumps and the retracted nipple. I underwent breast conservation surgery on December 5, 2014, following which the nipple retraction was corrected. The initial post-surgery biopsy report on 17th December did not show any cancer. I heaved a huge sigh of relief. I thought the danger had passed as I had been terribly worried all this time that this was the end of the road for me.

I was concerned about my children, getting them married and settled in life. My family members, too, had been anxious with the same thoughts.Everyone equated cancer with death. As I was recovering from the surgery, I noticed that my husband seemed upset one day and was crying. He told me with tears in his eyes that, based on the biopsy report, the surgeon had recommended removing the right breast. These words shook me, and only a woman can understand what I felt then. Now, I not only had cancer but also the very essence of femininity was going to be altered. All seemed dark, and it took me some time to process my thoughts and come to terms with the decision. In my rational mind, I knew that this was, of course, the right course of treatment.

However, I did accept the fact and composed myself before facing the family. I knew I had to be the strongest person now. If I broke down, my family members would lose their courage too. I spoke positively to them. I told them even with the diagnosis of cancer, God has provided a way out through this surgery. My chances of being cancer-free are very high, and I will be there to see the children get married and start their families and look after and nurture my grandchildren as well. There was so much to look forward to in life. That is when I realized the importance of having a positive outlook. Not only the person with cancer but also those around them benefit from a positive approach. The surgery was scheduled for December 21, 2014, and I remember my husband and family standing around as I was being wheeled into the operation theater. Once inside the theater, as the anesthetist was starting the intravenous line, I noticed the surgeons intently reviewing an X-ray film, and they seemed to be discussing something worriedly. They finally informed my family that a white spot on my ultrasound led them to suspect cancer had spread to the liver. They wanted to postpone the surgery till they were able to reassess my condition.

Initially, they did not tell me the reason for the postponement, and there were a thousand thoughts whirling around in my mind. However, my husband did tell me in a few days, and as advised, I underwent a PET CT scan.

This scan basically detects the presence of cancer cells anywhere in the body. The test result was expected on December 27, and the whole family and I waited anxiously for the results. The entire family, including my sisters and in-laws, was praying fervently for a favorable report. Each day seemed like an eternity. It was such a huge relief when we got the results. It was a false alarm; cancer had not spread anywhere else. The whole family celebrated the good news with me. I think it was after a long time that everyone in the family ate properly and slept well. My surgery date was now rescheduled. I opted to be operated on December 31 because I wanted the New Year to begin on a good note. I finally underwent a complete mastectomy on December 31, 2014. I also had complete lymph node dissection from the right axilla. My elder son, who lived in Ghaziabad, came to see me.

So far, we hadn't told my younger son about my diagnosis as he was still studying in Chennai and had one more semester to complete. Following the surgery, my mind cleared a bit. I felt I was winning this fight against cancer. My hope was being slowly restored, and I prepared myself to go forward. I was scheduled for six cycles of chemotherapy, and I had my first cycle of chemotherapy on January 21, 2015. I recovered well enough to attend a wedding in the family a few days later. No one at the gathering would have guessed I had undergone chemo. I think it was my extraordinary willpower that helped me carry it off. My extended family had not been told of my diagnosis. I did not want to be subjected to inquisitive stares and strange looks from people when they heard about the mastectomy. I was still in a fragile frame of mind and decided to take my time before sharing my story. A couple of weeks following the first chemo, I started experiencing hair loss. Although I was informed about this side-effect and thought I was mentally prepared to face it, I was still horrified on seeing my hair come out in huge clumps. My mother-in-law advised me not to worry about it too much and ignore it. That was good advice. When I lost all my hair, I glanced at myself in the mirror and could not believe what I was seeing.

I looked frightful, and I used to break down in tears. Hair is the crowning glory for a woman, and the loss is definitely hard to take. My face looked strange without my hair, and I lost my eyebrows too. People advised me that once the chemotherapy was completed, my hair would grow back thicker and healthier. This is my message as well to anyone who is undergoing chemo and is experiencing hair loss. Your hair does grow back better than it was before. But while on treatment, you do not have to feel bad and confine yourself to the house. You can invest in colorful scarves to wear while you are out. And if scarves are not comfortable for you, there are a lot of choices in wigs. Investing in a good wig that suits you is one of the best decisions you can make. It will boost your confidence and help you carry on your daily work.

My chemotherapy cycles continued. As I went to the hospital for each of my sessions, I got acquainted with a few people who were also coming in at the same time for their chemo. We would talk to each other and encourage each other. Each one of us undergoing chemotherapy had our own unique battle to fight, and none of us could lose hope. I made it a point to carefully follow all my doctor's instructions about medicines, diet, and exercise. Experiment and find out what food suits you and the days you are comfortable consuming them. For instance, for about five to six days immediately after a chemo cycle, you may be able to eat only bland and easily digestible food. I was in no rush and took each day as it came. I only wanted to get completely alright and healthy. I was advised not to go out in the daytime during the chemotherapy period. This is because the chemo medicines can make your skin sensitive and cause sunburn and allergies on exposure.

If you do have to go out, use sunscreen with SPF above 50 from a reputed brand. I was even taught some massaging exercises for my hand by the physiotherapist. These exercises were necessary to prevent my arm from swelling up.

My chemotherapy came to an end in August 2015, and the next phase of treatment commenced. I underwent 15 sessions of radiation therapy.

Later, hormone therapy was proposed once the radiation doses were over. It is still continuing. Today I am healthy, and my hair has grown back beautifully.

The motive behind sharing my story is to assure everyone out there that cancer is not an incurable disease. It is definitely curable if detected early. In fact, unlike diabetes and hypertension, it is not a lifelong condition once you are cured.

Do not be negligent about any symptoms in your body, be it a lump in the breast or anything else. Get yourself checked regularly. If I had been negligent in treating my disease, perhaps I would not be here to tell my story. To be honest, I have only one complaint. The swelling in my right hand bothers me sometimes. Because the lymph nodes were removed from my right axilla, I have a condition called lymphedema of the hand. It can be controlled to a large extent with exercises and massage, but still, there is some swelling. I do cry about that. After all, I am a woman, and physical appearance is important to me. My old clothes do not fit me, and I have to customize new clothes by making the right sleeves bigger than the left. However, I have made my peace with that now. It is a small price to pay for a cancer-free life. I have solved the problem of sleeves for the most part by switching over to sleeveless clothes. My message to everyone who has been diagnosed with cancer or is undergoing treatment would be as follows:

- Follow all the instructions of your doctors.
- Take your medicines regularly, check your diet, and do not neglect the exercises advised by your health team.

You can also take up other activities as your health permits, like yoga, meditation, and short walks. All these activities help build positivity, which is very important in this battle against cancer. It is very important to realize you can't do it alone. Take the help of all those around you who are willing to stand beside you. You will be surprised how many people want to help. I was blessed to have my husband's strong support throughout my treatment journey.

My husband's family was incredibly supportive too. They did not let me feel any kind of dearth, whether emotionally, physically, or financially. My neighbors, too, stood by me and gave me moral support and encouragement. This circle of love and support ensured that I could focus on my treatment. Along with the doctors, I am indebted to my family and friends, who lent their unconditional support throughout my treatment. It is commonly said that doctors are equal to Gods. This is not an exaggeration. Next to the Almighty, your doctor is a person who looks after your interests with utmost devotion and care. That is why I plead with you to believe what your doctor says. They know the best and no one else. Don't listen to others and lose hope.

I repeat: CANCER IS CURABLE! Read my story and be convinced.

Keep a positive outlook and have faith in your doctors.

Name: Anita Lal
Age: Undisclosed
Place: Lucknow

Before I share my experience as a breast cancer survivor, I would like my readers to think about some of the most annoying doubts. Doesn't a person have a life before the arrival of breast cancer?

And then, will you not have a life once this dreadful disease leaves you? My answer to these two questions will be pragmatic enough to impart a little positivity to the prevailing thought process among cancer patients. Remember, you had a life before cancer and will still have one, albeit a more experienced life, after you overcome this arduous battle. In fact, you will live till you are destined to live.

In my experience, breast cancer is like any other disease. It is like being involved in a terrible accident: unwarranted and unwanted.

I would say, breast cancer is like one of the worst nightmares. Being able to disclose one's good and bad experiences with the disease helps in nourishing better physical and mental well-being.

Sharing experiences helps in improving a patient's or survivor's emotional strength. It helps in an overall improvement in personal confidence. Why is breast cancer so appalling? Breast cancer therapy was quite expensive in the last century. And the cure rate was not that great either. It did not matter whether you were rich or poor; the treatment options were limited.

However, the situation is different now. Breast cancer is one of the most researched diseases and a wide variety of treatment procedures are now made possible. The scope of treatment is simple and is readily available in both government and private hospitals.

On the same note, with the increase and availability of diagnostic techniques and treatment, the number of patients has also increased. According to the KGMU statistics, the number of patients treated on a single day is 100 percent more than the number of doctors and the hospital staff capability. And to my surprise, about 80 percent of the patients are cured completely.

Nevertheless, I am not penning down my experience to talk about the success rates at KGMU. I wish to state the significance of breast cancer diagnosis and treatment within my tribe. Be it womanhood or motherhood, a woman is identified through her breasts. Yes, it does sound revolting but it is a brutal fact of our life. The breast is perceived as an emblem of motherhood, and it seems that the motherly instincts to love and cherish vanish once the breasts are gone. Under the present patriarchal societal norms, a woman is considered a machine to procreate. That's all! It's appalling but it's true. I was diagnosed with invasive ductal carcinoma of the left breast. In my condition, the cancer was present in the milk-producing ducts of the breast. Thus, you can see the plight that breast cancer can bring to motherhood.

I initially underwent chemotherapy, followed by total removal of the breast and later, radiation therapy to the chest wall. I am cured of cancer.

We live in a society that harbors a preconceived notion about a woman's role and necessity. A woman and her needs come at the lowest priority in society. Who bothers about her health?

Even in the twenty-first century, 50 percent of women suffer from gender inequality. Her life is designed to take care of others and not her own. No? The ordeal doesn't stop there. A woman must keep her beauty secured. She should epitomize the essence of beauty come what may. Don't we see the rise in cesarean delivery? Don't we hear about women worrying about the size and shape of their breasts? Why? Because we have been taught that women need to be perfect to keep the men happy and ensure that they succeed in bringing the next generation into the world. In short, more than a woman's brain, her breast is important for society. Her ability to reproduce makes her a complete woman. And honestly, all such detailed definition often comes from another woman. Have you wondered why? Because over the years, the patriarchal system has nourished our mental make-up too. Women often tend to think through a man's perspective and not their own. Shouldn't we mark this kind of thinking as racist? An inflexible notion against the whole woman race.

In my fight against cancer, I have learned profound lessons. Each cancer patient has her own set of challenges. Some patients were financially unstable, while others had no willpower to fight the disease despite having every kind of luxury in life.

As a cancer survivor, I would urge every cancer patient to be patient with the disease.

Pray for your cure, but do not keep banging your head over the disease; that will not help you in any way. You'll only end up lowering your self-esteem in the process. That's all. Cancer not only affects the body but also the mind. The only way to combat the disease is by not losing patience. However, we each have our own limitations, and not everyone can put on a brave face.

My intention behind this note is singular: to encourage every woman to come out of their cocoon of self-deprecation. A woman's worth is beyond her beauty and physical features. Breasts are as significant as any other organ in a woman's body. Just like how one cannot breathe with a blocked nose and must get it treated, a woman must not keep calm with a disease like breast cancer. If the disease can be cured by removing the breasts, one must go ahead. After all, a healthy life is more valuable than a beautiful body.

Cancer is frightening, but with the advent of newer technologies, it is curable. One must hold on to courage and perseverance. No societal barriers or obsolete temperament should hinder the treatment process. Lastly, womanhood is beautiful in itself; whether one enjoys motherhood or not is immaterial to the spirit of womanhood. More than being a disease, breast cancer induces a kind of phobia; nevertheless, one must come forward to get diagnosed at an early stage and start the treatment regimen. Women are not machines to procreate. They are beautiful souls to be taken care of. I would request all to go for a thorough check-up whenever the need arises. There is indeed a correlation between womanhood, motherhood, and breast cancer. But when it is about leading a healthy life, every ingredient carries a separate identity, where getting rid of cancer must become the prime focus.

Do not let cancer conquer your mind.

Social stigma is often the major reason in India for delaying medical consultation. Misconceptions regarding the disease and the patriarchal nature of the society, especially in a rural setting where women are more dependent on men for their health needs, may lead to such stigma. There is an absolute and urgent requirement for early diagnosis and management of breast cancer. There is a sizeable number of breast cancer patients who are facing a delay in diagnosis and treatment, which stems from the lack of awareness and resources, wrong perception of the disease by the patients, and poor physician approach.

The after-effects of cancer treatment, such as loss of hair, resected breasts, open or healed wounds, and other physical deformities, make it more unacceptable and prone to stigma. These physical changes become near normal with time after completion of treatment.

The hair does grow back, and it can be more beautiful than before, as narrated by Mrs. Anju.

As healthcare professionals, we always attempt to make the lives of breast cancer patients easier by reducing all forms of the stigma associated with it. Stigma carries a heavy emotional burden that can be mitigated better through the involvement of the family. On a similar note, awareness programs may not treat the disease but can certainly help in eliminating the myths and the tag of 'social taboo.' The root of the problem goes down to the lack of knowledge.

I would like to stress that breast cancer is a curable disease. Early diagnosis is the key to a better and more favorable outcome. Consider breast cancer just as you would any other illness and not as a taboo subject. This is the first step to giving women a better deal. Men and women need to be encouraged to talk about women's health concerns without inhibitions. Only then can we succeed in removing the stigma associated with breast cancer. We must work to increase awareness about timely medical consultations and breast self-examination. **Abandon the stigma associated with breast cancer!**

2

WOMEN'S HEALTH IS UNIVERSALLY IGNORED

A healthy woman makes a healthy family

Women are the building blocks of the family. Though often they are relegated to the background, they play a major role in holding intact the fabric of family life. Women play a prominent role in the provision of healthcare for their families. Apart from being nurturers and caregivers, mothers are the first teachers to their children. Maternal illness is said to affect children adversely. Healthy women are said to be the cornerstone of a healthy society. The International Council on Women's Health Issues (ICOWHI) is an international nonprofit association that is dedicated to promoting the healthcare and well-being of women and girls throughout the world, through participation, empowerment, advocacy, education, and research[1].

---

[1] https://www.ncbi.nlm.nih.gov/pmc/articles/PMC3703826/

In their white paper on women's health issues, they state that women and girls have specific health needs, and those are not currently being met by the health systems they are under. ICOWHI states that to improve the health, healthcare, and well-being of women and girls, a concerted and integrated effort has to be made in identifying specific areas of need, promoting education, getting over socio-cultural norms, improving economic conditions to provide economic independence, and empowering women to make their own decisions with regard to their health. The health of families and communities can be said to be tied to the health of the woman. Women's health can be improved by educating them, empowering them, and addressing the various health issues they face at different times of their lives. Educating the woman is equivalent to educating the family. A healthy woman will ensure a healthy family, and healthy families make healthy communities and nations.

Traditionally, a woman's health has always been underplayed and not been given importance equal to what a man receives. The man's role has always been perceived as that of provider and protector, and hence his health and well-being are assumed to warrant more attention and care.

Women's health was initially never given much importance in our country. In our society, women have been conditioned to be extremely patient and silent about their health issues. Why do women suffer in silence? The answer lies in their upbringing. From childhood, a girl is taught to follow the prevailing societal norms. And these norms dictate that a woman's role is to look after her family, which includes her husband, children, and any other male member residing in the home. Self-care is a totally alien concept to her. The typical Indian woman has been portrayed as reclusive and shy, and these qualities have been glorified. In reality, though, the woman often suffers from neglect and low self-esteem. She is uninformed and ignorant about her health, which prevents her from seeking medical help. Women in India face numerous issues related to health and well-being: malnutrition, poor maternal health, sexually transmitted diseases, breast cancer, domestic violence, etc.

In certain societies, most of the attention and care is focused on the male children or the men in general. The best of the food is served to them, with the women making do with the leftovers. Still, in certain sections of society, there is inequality in power and independence between the genders when it comes to decision-making in matters relating to health, just as it exists in all other spheres, such as education and career choice. Every educational effort should be taken to remove this taboo from society.

Many women who suffer from severe pain during their menstrual cycles are said to have 'periods pain.' Women experience mood changes during this period, and they may be termed as moody, cranky, hypochondriacal, or even hysterical. It is interesting to note that, in earlier times, the uterus was believed to be the cause of a woman's symptoms. It is unfortunate that many of these beliefs still exist in some stratum of society. It is true that hormones do play a large role in the health of women, but it is always important to look into other causes of her ailment.

Women should neither neglect their symptoms nor face discrimination in the family. They should get access to and benefit from quality healthcare. To address these issues, what is needed is education and empowerment. The importance of the health of women needs to be voiced. Women need to be educated about their roles in society, the consequences of neglecting their health, the importance of good nutrition, the importance of seeking early medical help, and the benefits of self-care.

Role of Women in Society

Women have long been relegated to the roles of caretakers and nurturers in the family. Throughout their lifetime, they may don the different mantles of a daughter, sister, daughter-in-law, mother, etc.

Whatever the position they may occupy, their main occupation would be caring for the family. In traditional Indian society, the girl child is taught a totally different set of values from what a boy would be taught.

The girls are taught to be homely, submissive, timid, and obedient. They are told that their aspirations should be to become ideal wives and mothers. The main role they would play would be that of a home-maker. As a daughter, the girl child is expected to care for her parents. Most of the time, she is not allowed to make her own decisions.

When she gets married, her role becomes more demanding. She is now expected to look after her husband and his family as well. With the arrival of children, her responsibilities increase greatly and she is left with no time for herself.

As a mother, she is in the unique position of looking after all the needs of her children. She is now responsible for all their food and clothing. She is their first teacher. Nurturing a child from infancy to adulthood is quite a long process and the best years of her life are devoted to this task. In reality, women play a very crucial role in society. They are responsible for the upbringing of the next generation of adults.

As the burden of caregiving keeps increasing, the woman loses interest in herself. She always gives priority to her family's needs and ignores her own requirements, including her health and nutritional needs. Women should be taught the importance of looking after themselves. Only if they are healthy, can they effectively take care of their family.

Importance of Self-Care

The World Health Organization defines self-care as "the ability of families, individuals, and communities to promote health, prevent disease, maintain health, and cope with illness or disability with or without the support of a healthcare provider." In simple terms, it means you take care of yourself to remain healthy and accomplish all you want to do.

Self-care includes anything you do to keep yourself healthy— physically, mentally, or spiritually. Women neglect to take proper care of themselves for a number of reasons:

1. Responsibilities and burdens: As a woman cares for her growing family, she often finds that she does not have sufficient time to devote to her own needs.
2. Social conditioning: Traditionally, women have been taught that their role as caregivers is more important than looking after themselves.
3. Do not want undue attention: Women do not want to draw any undue attention to themselves by voicing their needs. This is the inherent nature of most women.
4. Lack of knowledge: Illiteracy and ignorance about the health issues in women can be cause for neglect.
5. Financial dependency: Women are generally dependent on their menfolk for all their needs, including their health needs. This could be a deterrent in looking after themselves. They can be hesitant to approach the husband or the head of the family for money.

    This lack of self-care can have serious consequences on the well-being of women. When women neglect their health needs, not only do they end up having serious physical ailments, but they also have associated mental and emotional problems.

Let us look at some of the effects of not having proper self-care in women.

1. Anger and Impatience: When you are overworked and stressed, you do not spend enough time on yourself. This stress can make you short-tempered and impatient.
2. Low energy levels: Lack of proper rest and relaxation can make you feel like you are constantly running on empty. You feel like you are in a permanent state of exhaustion.
3. Feeling of hopelessness: It is important to take some time out of your busy day for some activity that you enjoy doing. It should not involve taking care of others. This will give you a positive outlook on life.

4. Symptoms of headache and stomach ache: These are all symptoms relating to stress. You will often find that these symptoms disappear when you take time out for yourself.

5. Depression and Anxiety: These are slightly more serious issues related to lack of self-care. If you think you are experiencing these symptoms, it is important that you seek professional help immediately.

6. Sleep disturbances: When you are stressed out, you may experience difficulties in falling asleep. Or you may have a disturbed sleep pattern. For proper sleep, your mind has to be at rest.

7. Brain fog: Altered sleep patterns and stress can lead to decreased mental alertness and concentration.

8. Weight gain: Lack of self-care includes making poor nutritional choices. You may choose to eat comfort foods over a healthy diet. This is because comfort foods can make you feel happy, and they are also easily accessible. This can lead to unhealthy weight gain.

9. Avoidance of health issues: Lack of self-care eventually results in neglecting even serious health problems. When you do not seek medical help at the right time, many diseases can have lasting sequelae or consequences. When treated early most illnesses are curable.

10. Avoiding society: When you are tired and depressed, it follows that you will not want to meet others socially or enjoy the company of relatives and friends. Your social contacts will decrease slowly.

Self-care, as I mentioned earlier, involves taking time to look after your physical, mental, and emotional/spiritual health. It can be called a wholesome health routine. There are many ways in which you can take care of yourself. It basically involves recognizing that you as a person are of great importance to your family, and you can give the best of yourself only if you are in good shape. It is as important for you to have enough rest as any other member of the family.

It is very important to remember that self-care is NOT selfish and do not feel guilty about taking time for yourself. In fact, when you are healthy in body, mind, and soul, you can take better care of the others in your family. Self-care is not an expensive business. Do whatever makes you happy. Spend some time every day pursuing your interests or hobbies.

Ensure that you take your meals on time and eat healthy food, not leftovers. Make sure to get proper rest, and keep your resting time sacrosanct. Regular exercise goes a long way in keeping the body and mind healthy.

Go for a walk daily, even if it is just a half-hour stroll on your terrace. It can also help avoid excessive weight gain. Any illness or problems should be addressed immediately. If you feel something is wrong or there is pain somewhere, make an appointment with your doctor for a check-up.

If visiting friends or relatives is a stressbuster for you, ensure that you take time out for such visits. Keep in touch with old friends. Also, it is equally important that you stay away from anyone who causes you stress.

When you take care of ourself, you build resilience to withstand any stress. You can easily bounce back from any trauma or stressful situation. It has been clinically proved that self-care can reduce or eliminate symptoms of anxiety and depression. It improves your concentration and increases your happiness. You give yourself a chance to step aside and breathe. You can avoid burnout. It not only improves physical energy and stamina but also your focus and mental acuity. It keeps your energy levels high and helps you perform your duties better.

Following a healthy lifestyle not only minimizes the chance of illness but also helps in identifying any disease condition early. This includes the diagnosis of cancer as well.

Early diagnosis of any disease means a better chance of cure. When you are happy, there is less frustration and anger, and this can ultimately lead to a happy family life.

Importance of Regular Health Check-Up

A health check-up can allow the doctor to pick up signs of an illness that you are not even aware of having. This is especially true in the case of breast cancer. Let me tell you about some of the benefits of going for a regular health consultation.

1. A regular health check-up can help in the detection of diseases early before complications set in.
2. Early detection of a disease condition means early treatment and a better chance of cure or recovery.
3. Regular health check-up allows keeping track of the health status. It will give access to vital information that helps monitor physical, mental, and emotional health so that timely actions can be taken.
4. Healthcare costs are reduced when a disease is detected early.
5. Going for a regular health check-up provides an opportunity to build a good relationship with the doctor or healthcare provider. This will ensure that you can tell your problems without hesitancy, and the doctor too will be able to communicate more effectively with you. This paves the way for efficient medical management and treatment.
6. A good doctor will encourage you to be proactive and take the right steps to stay healthy. They will give you tips on how to maintain good habits and an overall healthy lifestyle.

Consequences of Delayed Treatment

I have talked about the importance of early diagnosis. Small problems can quickly blow up and progress if not treated on time. Delay in treatment causes additional stress on the individual, the family, the treating doctor, and the healthcare system. The treatment becomes expensive and may even require an emergency operation.

In advanced breast cancer, operations are never possible and the outcome becomes poorer. Women often delay seeking treatment for their health issues because of lack of awareness, financial constraints, inaccessibility of healthcare, etc.

Challenges That I See in My Practice

In my years of medical practice, I have seen a lack of self-care. This may be because women have been programmed to think less of themselves and more about their families, especially the male members of the family. They spend all their time and energy looking after others. Some of the other reasons for not seeking early medical care, especially with respect to breast cancer, that I have encountered are listed below:

Healthcare-Related Factors

There may be unavailability of good healthcare facilities in a nearby place. All the government sector hospitals do not have separate diagnostic or treatment facilities for breast cancer. All patients with breast-related problems have to go and meet the doctor in the common OPD areas in these hospitals. Healthcare facilities are heterogeneous in distribution and many hospitals have inadequate cancer treatment infrastructure. There are limited radiation facilities in many states. For instance, the diagnostic facilities are not in one place but rather spread out throughout the hospital.

This makes it more difficult for the patients to get all their investigations done. There is also overcrowding, which can be a deterrent in bringing women to the hospital.

Patient-Related Factors

There is an inborn hesitancy in women to share their health problems with anyone, let alone a doctor.

Often, the women want to consult only a female physician. The absence of a female doctor in the nearest health facility is one of the reasons why women do not seek medical help early. There is a fear that once their health condition is known, they may be isolated by their family. In general, women have low awareness of the various diseases that can affect them, and that includes breast cancer as well. They are hesitant to undergo any investigations, especially biopsies, fearing the worst.

In some instances, they do not want to accept the diagnosis and go from one doctor to another hoping for a favorable verdict. This causes a delay in the start of treatment. Even after the correct diagnosis is made after consultation with a specialist at a reputed hospital, they sometimes resort to alternative medical therapies.

Many women discontinue the treatment once started due to a lack of motivation or other family causes. Women give a lot of importance to what their other relatives, friends, and neighbors have to say. Various home remedies are tried before seeking proper medical help. They try to follow the advice of all, but this actually hampers and delays the right treatment.

Social Factors

Women are socially indoctrinated to ignore their health. This results in a delay in consulting a physician. Women's health is commonly neglected in families. Women delay seeking medical help often because they are not financially independent. They fear they might drain the family's finances.

The male members of the family are generally unconcerned about the health of the women and do not get involved in their welfare.

Disease-Related Factors

Breast cancer invokes inevitable fear of all types of suffering and a feeling of helplessness. It is understandable and cannot be removed.

By reassuring our patients, we can boost their morale and confidence. The prolonged treatment required to combat breast cancer is a major deterrent in its therapy. Very often, women think that the cost would be unaffordable and would drain the family's resources badly. When there are no cancer specialists to treat breast cancer close by, women choose not to get treated. The long trips required for each consultation and each therapy session make them give up on their treatment.

SURVIVOR NOTES

Alka was diagnosed to have breast cancer in 2016 and is a conqueror. She underwent surgery followed by chemotherapy and radiotherapy. She is now cured of cancer and her life is an inspiration for newer cancer patients. Her story highlights the importance of self-care and seeking treatment for cancer symptoms without delay.

Name: Alka Agarwal
Age: 34 years
Place: Lucknow

I am Alka Agarwal, a resident of Lucknow, Uttar Pradesh. I am 34 years old and married. My husband, Pankaj Agarwal, runs a small business in the Yahiyaganj wholesale market in Lucknow. He is a trader of Pooja Pats or Bajots. These are the small platforms made out of wood, aluminum, or silver, used to keep idols of Gods.

Our home is close to Yahiyaganj as well. As a homemaker, my life has always revolved around my husband, two children, and home. I have a son and a daughter who are both studying in a nearby secondary school. My son is 14 years old, and he is in the 9th standard, while my daughter is just 11 and studies in class 5.

The year 2016 has been the most memorable year of my life, though not in a good sense. I can easily call it the gloomiest year in our lives. I will never forget September 2016, when I got the earth-shattering diagnosis of breast cancer. As soon as the diagnosis was confirmed, every aisle of life seemed to come under the darkest clouds of grief and sickness. My family didn't know whether to grieve or fear, where to move forward, or whom to approach.

Cancer is not something palatable. For me especially, it was a time of great regret as I bitterly lamented my negligence. Why? Because I had felt a very small lump in my left breast some six months before. I still remember to have felt the lump while dressing up. Initially, I remained anxious for a couple of days and still did not mention it to my family. There was no pain, and it did not hinder my daily activities. Days passed by doing my regular chores, and I had completely forgotten about the lump.

Five months later, I suddenly realized that the lump had grown slightly bigger. But there was still no pain or no other discomfort. I continued to remain silent and did not share this fact with anyone else. Over the next 20 to 25 days, I noticed the lump size gradually increasing. And I had started feeling a tightness in my breast when I bent down to do my usual household activities. A mild niggling pain used to crop up while working at home. I was anxious about the increasing discomfort, but I continued to keep this a secret. Today, I can blatantly reveal that it was the biggest mistake I had ever made.

By the time I could even think about the lump, Navarathri had arrived. It was a great time of festivity in our city. For my husband, too, it was a peak season for sales. Pooja items are usually in maximum demand at this time. As the festival days came nearer, my husband was working long hours, and he used to leave home early for his shop and would return quite late in the evening.

I finally decided to do something about my problem. On the first day of Navarathri, I finished all my household chores and went to a clinic in the evening. It was near my home, and the lady doctor was a well-known gynecologist in Lucknow, and lots of women from our area used to visit her for all their health issues.

I was extremely nervous as I sat in the waiting room for my token number to be called. After examination, the doctor was furious seeing the large size of the lump. She kept asking why I had not gotten it checked earlier but assured me that it could be cured. She advised some tests and mammography. In the evening, I informed my husband. He, too, sounded positive and lent me some encouraging words.

"You should have told me sooner," he said. The very next day, I underwent mammography and the blood tests. We again consulted the doctor with the mammogram report. After seeing the report, she asked me to wait outside as she spoke to my husband. I was very nervous sitting in the waiting room. Somehow, I had a hunch that it was going to be cancer.

The doctor did reveal to my husband that I had cancer. She advised him to consult a specialist for further treatment. It must have been quite a shock for my husband. After all, he had come to know about my breast lump only the previous day, and here today, the diagnosis was cancer in the breast. But he took it with good grace. He tried to protect me and never told me exactly what the doctor had told him. After a day of thinking and planning, my husband started asking all his trader friends and his relatives about where to go for further treatment.

Many people gave references and suggestions. Some people even shared positive stories about how their relatives had recovered from breast cancer with a positive outcome. All these words encouraged me greatly, and my fear slowly subsided. My brother-in-law recommended that I should go to King George's Medical University (KGMU), Lucknow, for a consultation. He told us that the institute had reputed doctors who had successfully treated many breast cancer patients. So, that is how we came to meet Dr. Anand Mishra at KGMU. He saw my test results and mammogram report. He advised me to do a few more tests and a PET CT. After going through all my test reports, he confirmed that I was suffering from breast cancer Stage 3 and told us the steps of management. Chemotherapy was the first treatment option, followed by surgery.

He was very encouraging, and his words gave a lot of mental strength to both my husband and me. I mentally prepared myself for the complete treatment. Chemotherapy was started on the very next day. I will never forget the day of my first chemo; I was still in the middle of my Navarathri fasting. The first chemotherapy session coincided with my fasting for Ashtami. I had heard about hair loss following chemotherapy. The doctor too cautioned me about it. Loss of hair saddened me a little as I had long and luxurious hair. However, the medical staff at the hospital consoled me saying my hair would grow back once chemotherapy was completed. And most likely, it would grow back thicker and better. It was more important to start the battle against cancer immediately. I decided in my mind that I would win this fight and get well soon. I had three cycles of chemo before my surgery and three cycles following my surgery. I had a complete left mastectomy with axillary node clearance. Later, I underwent 27 days of radiation therapy. My final radiation therapy session was on January 24, 2017. It was a huge relief to complete all the treatment.

I understand that my whole breast was removed as I had an advanced tumor. If only I had been more health-conscious and taken medical advice as soon as I had first noticed the lump, I probably would not have had to undergo removal of the breast.

However, I am thankful that I have been able to cross this path and come out successful. I want to tell everyone, "Never neglect a breast lump." Please see your doctor immediately. Many lumps are indeed harmless, but let the specialists make that decision. Breast cancer, if detected early, is completely curable. The chances of a long and healthy cancer-free life are so much higher when the disease is diagnosed and treated in the early stages. That is why it is important to check every lump and start therapy early.

I am healthy now and leading a normal life. I am grateful to my doctors for the encouragement. Dr. Anand was a big source of hope and encouragement. My only concern these days is the swelling in my left hand. It is due to lymph collection as the lymph nodes have been removed in the left arm. I am slowly learning to live with it. I diligently do all the arm exercises taught by the physiotherapist.

I am hoping someday my arm will also return to normal. My family, too, stood by me through the whole ordeal. My husband and children were pillars of support, especially during the difficult days of chemotherapy. My sister-in-law, too, was a huge support. She took over all my household chores and did not let me do any work throughout my treatment period. She wanted me to focus only on my recovery. The care and concern shown by my doctors and my family helped me to fight against cancer. As a cancer survivor, I urge every woman to concentrate on her health.

Do not neglect any change in your body, especially the breasts.

As a doctor practicing in India, I would confirm that there are several factors involved in making common people ignore their health issues.

On a professional front, I have been seeing India's healthcare system battling various issues, including the low number of institutions compared to the number of cancer patients seeking treatment. There is a lack of well-equipped medical institutes and training facilities for cancer treatment in the government sector in many cities.

Moreover, the hesitance is more pronounced when patients with breast cancer do not find a separate OPD to discuss their problems. Our cultural norms somehow make women shy of talking about their breasts and private parts. And, as the first step in diagnosing breast cancer is the examination of the breasts, a general OPD seems frightening. The apprehension is compounded when women do not find female doctors to examine them.

Prateeksha is a breast cancer survivor, and her story also highlights the importance of self-care. She helps several new breast cancer patients navigate the course of treatment in our support group.

Name: Prateeksha Pandey
Age: 34, Unmarried
Place: Lucknow

My name is Prateeksha Pandey, and I am here to unveil my experience as a cancer survivor. I was diagnosed with cancer in January 2018. Everyone who knew me was shell-shocked and worried. In fact, my father fell ill once he knew about my diagnosis.

I am inherently an optimistic person. I never get bogged down and prefer to look at the positive aspects of life all the time. I requested all my friends and family to send only positive vibes. People known to me were so scared that my best friend had stopped talking to me. She could not fathom how to console me.

On the other hand, I was mentally prepared and convinced her that everything would be fine. As I narrate my experience, I would like to motivate all people living with cancer to be positive.

I faced the most brutal truth of cancer when I realized how insignificant women's health in our society is. The journey is difficult, but there is indeed a trouble-free destination. Willpower and positive thoughts are the strongest weapons against cancer. In the beginning, I had encountered so many people who harnessed the negative effects of cancer treatment. Some even declared that cancer patients could survive only for six months after the operation. Honestly, I was okay with six months too. I did not wish to 'die' before dying. I wanted to live happily in whatever time was left to me. Initially, when I met my doctor for the first time at KGMU, I asked him about my chances of survival. He convincingly assured me that I could be cured. I was also introduced during that visit to a number of cancer survivors and was assured of the success rate of the treatment. I underwent a series of tests for confirmation of the diagnosis.

Soon, I was admitted to the hospital. The whole day, some relative or friend used to pay me a visit. I never felt like a patient at all, and never did I ask anyone to spend a night in the hospital with me. I consulted the doctor over the sequence of treatment. I wished to know if I could proceed with chemotherapy first and then opt for an operation. I was even concerned if my breasts would be removed. As per the diagnosis and staging of the disease, the doctor admitted that my breast could not be conserved completely. On hearing this prognosis, I opted to undergo the operation first and it was scheduled for February 2, 2018. Somehow, I was never scared of the disease. I always believed that everything would come to normal soon. God must have sent me into this world with a purpose. My operation was successful and I was sent home. Most of my family members were supportive, but I was able to see through to the true intentions of a few of them. Their attitude toward me had changed. Initially, it did hurt me; however, I soon realized that I was self-sufficient. This bad phase probably served to make me realize the same.

My father and sister used to visit me. Still, she had her own familial responsibilities. My treatment was going to be a long one, so I asked them to visit as and when they got time. I did not want to bother anyone. I started my chemotherapy on March 9, 2018. The only thing that bothered me was the impending loss of my long and beautiful plaits of hair. A woman's beauty is often ratified by her breasts and beautiful hair. And now, I would soon lose both. Another disastrous news set in during my second chemotherapy session. My sister's son used to call me often; however, I did not receive a call from him that day. It was unusual and I called to enquire. My sister simply said that she was busy cooking and would call later. However, when I reached home, I got the crushing news. I could not believe my ears. My nephew had passed away. Words failed me, and I just cannot describe my sister's plight; how terrible it is for a mother to hold her son's dead body! My sister used to be so fragile, and still, she did not wish to bother me during the chemo with such awful news. I decided to go stay with her in Delhi.

People did try to stop me as I was not well enough, but I could not leave my sister alone at that moment. I came back to Lucknow for my third chemo and again went back to my sister. And on my way back, I faced another setback, another thorn in my path. My mother had suffered a brain hemorrhage, and she was counting her days. My whole day was spent traveling from one place to another. All of a sudden, I was fenced by so many challenges.

Along with my chemotherapy and its side effects, I had to take care of my mother, who was completely bedridden now. Along with my own deteriorating condition—fever, nausea, and all—I had to now take care of my filial responsibilities too. I kept my health issues under wraps and concentrated on my duties to my mother and the household. Once, during the course of treatment, I asked the doctor if I could go to work. The doctor smiled and said I was the first patient with whom he had to plead to take adequate rest. Usually, he would have to encourage the other patients to get back to their normal life, but I was completely the opposite. I was not at all interested in taking a break. However, my sister, father, and friends did a lot for me. Cancer treatment was painful, but their support and presence made me feel strong enough to combat the disease.

During the course of radiation, bathing was prohibited. The weather too was not conducive. Moreover, I had to finish my household chores and go for the radiation therapy session and again had to come back and resume my duties. I had got wounds here and there, and I had no route of escape. My radiation therapy was completed on August 29 and I went to be with my sister on September 2. My wounds were deep and painful. Deep down, I was depressed often. Sometimes, death seemed a better option than living like this. But then again, a slender voice would whisper within and urge me to live.

Within a few weeks, my wounds started to heal. In fact, I attended a National Conference in Jaipur and even participated in the walkathon. I had a wonderful experience in Jaipur. Everyone was so supportive and positive that I truly felt indebted to have gotten in touch with so many wonderful souls.

I never knew that a disease could bring such a positive influence on anyone. I had a marvelous experience with the volunteers. Somewhere, I could feel my life getting back to normalcy.

Similarly, I could see the true faces of so many people around. The one who promised to be by my side forever had almost forgotten my mere existence. My father always asked me to get a wig to restore my beauty. I never agreed. My sister used to wonder about my perseverance and often worried about my physical and emotional pain. She once declared that I had become an emotionless stone. However, my perspective was quite different. I had not turned harder, but I had become stronger than before. And with my consultant's initiative toward helping cancer patients, we all were getting closer to normalcy. Once in October, I went for a review to KGMU and then came back to Delhi. It so happened that I felt like talking to Rakha *Bhabhi*, one of the friends I had made during the conference. I called and received the awful news of her demise. My innards churned on hearing that news. I was so shattered that since that day, I have stopped calling anyone. A kind of fear grew within me. Whomever I called, I was told they had died. I just stopped making any calls, but would talk if anyone called.

I kept traveling. I would spend a fortnight with my sister and then visit my friends. I even went and participated in the Ayodhya program. I was a lot better now, and my pain and wounds had decreased. Still, I could never forget those horrendous days of radiation therapy. Yet, I was trying to follow my normal routine. Let me tell you about an interesting incident. I had a review on January 14 and I went to attend Kumbh Mela on the 17th. My 'crop-cut' hairstyle and the way I had dressed misled people into thinking that I was a government official. However, I just felt happy while helping them. Soon, Dr. Anand gave me a wonderful opportunity when I went to meet him for my follow-up in April 2018. He asked me to participate in a program to be held in Lucknow for cancer survivors. Participating in that program as a cancer survivor was a dream come true because I wished to help people who were suffering from cancer and were scared of the disease and its treatment.

I would like to thank everyone who helped me in my battle with cancer.

On the same note, my heartfelt gratitude goes to those who did not stand by my side as well. Their unsupportive nature actually made me self-sustaining. I shall be indebted to my doctor and his whole team for their unconditional support. My motive behind penning down my experience is to encourage people to speak out. I would like to urge every woman to identify the symptoms and get treated as soon as possible. Cancer patients should never lose their confidence. Always surround yourself with positive people and nurture good thoughts within you.

Secondly, I must confess that the treatment is not as expensive as people consider it to be. Doctors are competent with the latest technologies and help the patients in every way possible. I can assure everyone that good treatment is no longer restricted to big cities like Delhi or Mumbai. Even the small cities have excellent doctors to take care of cancer patients.

I apologize if my words have hurt anyone's sentiments. I have indeed received immense love and support from many of my loved ones. If the truth is told, a woman is bound to societal norms and restrictions right from her birth. Our health and welfare sink to the bottom of a family's priority list and our basic needs are often neglected. As I narrate my experience, I urge every woman to be vigilant toward her own health. We must not wait for others to take care of us. We must be available to ourselves. On the same note, every cancer survivor must come forward in support of other cancer victims. Lastly, never lose your willpower. The best weapon against cancer is the patient's willpower.

Your health is important too. Do not neglect it.

As you can see from Prateeksha's experience, a woman plays numerous roles in her lifetime and carries many burdens on her shoulder. This leads her to neglect her health.

In my practice, I have come across numerous women who gave priority to their family's needs and neglected their own. I tell them never to take their health for granted.

You have to make yourself a priority. Make time for yourself. Ensure that you get your health checked regularly. Ensure that you eat and sleep properly. And most importantly, please get any symptoms of breast lumps or changes checked out immediately.

In summary, I would say women's health plays a very important role in making a healthy society. Women's health is important because they are the building blocks of the family. They are the ones responsible for bringing the next generation into this world. Healthy women have healthy babies who grow into healthy adults. They are also the primary caregivers and nurturers in the family. To be healthy, the girl child and the woman have to be educated and empowered to take responsibility for their health. The importance of self-care needs to be taught. Women need to know that they cannot be everything to everyone all the time at the cost of self-neglect. Personal time out should be encouraged. The importance of early diagnosis and treatment must be made clear to them. This is especially true in the case of breast cancer, where early diagnosis and treatment ensure a high rate of complete cure. But is cancer treatment affordable to all? Let us talk about that in the next chapter.

3

FINANCIAL ASPECTS OF THE DISEASE

Cancer treatment is within your reach

The diagnosis of cancer definitely strikes fear in every heart. Of the myriad thoughts that swarm through the mind, one of the most pervading ones would be fear of the cost of treatment. A diagnosis of cancer is sure to bring numerous changes in a family. In the ensuing period of therapy, the role of the woman has to be taken over by others. There is a lot of disruption and adjusting in the family structure.

If it is a young mother who has breast cancer, then the care of her children would be on her mind. If there are old parents in the home, their care too is of concern. Over and above all these concerns, there is another thought looming through the mind: Can we afford the cost of treatment?

In addition to the deteriorating health and psychological stress, breast cancer patients and their families undergo economic distress, and due to the high cost of treatment and a lack of financial protection, they incur huge expenditures. The costs concerned with cancer therapy can be direct or indirect. Indirect costs are also called out-of-pocket expenditures. Aside from the actual cost of the medicines and chemo drugs used in the treatment, there are a lot of other expenses. It starts with transport. Traveling to and fro between hospital and home numerous times can notch up quite a bill.

The Government of India Railway Ministry provides concession on rail fares for cancer patients. Initial costs include consultation charges and investigation costs. The consultation can be done in government hospitals with a minimum registration charge. There are no bed charges, and the patients are provided free meals as well. Investigations are subsidized and done under various schemes. The cost of surgery is minimum. This holds true for King George's Medical University (KGMU) as well.

Although the treatment is free at government hospitals, if the person is a daily wage earner or if the husband is a small business owner, the loss of each day's wage or earnings adds up to the cost. The patient is not likely to go alone for a consultation, so the accompanying person also loses out. This may not seem like a big expense to those who are working in organizations where they can avail leave facilities or claim insurance coverage. But for a small-time business owner or a daily wage earner, this is indeed a big expense. This is one of the reasons why patients do not go to tertiary hospitals for cancer therapy in spite of the excellent treatment available there. The out-of-pocket expenditures are usually not covered by the insurance schemes.

Even the government schemes, such as the Ayushman Bharath Yojana, cover only the actual medical expenses. I have mentioned in the previous chapter that early-stage treatment is easy, less expensive, and less complicated with a high cure rate.

Financial Burden of Therapy

An article in the Economic Times a few years ago mentioned that a diagnosis of cancer could easily disrupt a family's finances due to the loss of a source of income.[2] A 2004 study on the economic burden of cancer on Indian households by Anup Karan et al. reported that the spending in a home with a cancer patient was 36 percent to 44 percent more than that in other households. These expenses were mainly transport costs, hospitalization charges, consultation visits, out-of-pocket spending, etc. Families in rural areas resort to selling their assets or borrowing from family and friends or moneylenders. Household costs also increase because there are many visitors. Let us see what the costs involved in the treatment of breast cancer are in detail:

1. **Cost of diagnosis:** The initial costs involved in the management of breast cancer are the costs of diagnosing the condition. These include the cost of consultation and the costs involved with investigations. Often patients go to multiple consultants before getting a correct diagnosis. A private consultation can easily cost anywhere from Rs 500 to Rs 1000. Investigations to diagnose breast cancer include FNAC, biopsy, ultrasonography of breast, and mammography. In advanced cases where the disease has spread, additional investigations, such as MRI and PET-CT, are called for.

2. **Cost of treatment:** This is one of the major costs for a cancer patient. This includes the cost of surgery, chemotherapy, and radiotherapy. Hospitalization costs can run up to many lakhs of rupees in private hospitals. And if any of these procedures result in side effects, they need to be managed, and this adds to the cost as well. Certain patients require targeted therapy or immunotherapy.

   These treatments are expensive and cannot be afforded by many people.

---

[2]https://economictimes.indiatimes.com/wealth/insure/can-you-bear-the-cost-of-cancer-treatment-find-out-how-to-buy-the-best-cover/articleshow/47744432.cms

3. **Loss of income:** If the woman was a working and earning member of the family before her diagnosis, the loss of her income can be a burden to the family. This holds true if the patient is self-employed or is a daily wage earner. Women in regular employment in the private sector or the government sector can avail sick leave facilities. Each time, a family member has to accompany the patient to the hospital for all the investigations and treatment procedures. Again, if this person, most likely the husband, is self-employed or a daily wage earner, he would lose his income too. The long treatment and missed days at work can lead to loss of business opportunities for those having small businesses of their own.

4. **Travel expense:** Specialist doctors and advanced investigation facilities are usually not available in villages, semi-urban, and rural areas. The patient has to travel to the diagnostic center to avail of these facilities. This may involve traveling numerous times to the city for various tests and investigations.

5. **Food and stay:** Traveling to a different town or city from your place of stay involves costs relating to food and stay as well. At times the patient might have to stay overnight or for a few days in the town or city. This can be expensive.

6. **Extra support:** If there are no family members to look after the children when a woman is diagnosed with breast cancer, she might have to hire extra help. This adds to the financial burden. Similarly, if he owns a small business, the husband will have to add to the staff to cover the days he has to accompany his wife for treatment.

7. **Repaying loans:** Often, when there is no insurance cover, families resort to taking loans from moneylenders or pawning their valuables for money to aid the treatment. Paying the interest on these loans is very taxing, especially with the loss of income.

Does this mean cancer therapy is totally unaffordable for people in the lower economic groups? Not at all. There are numerous resources available that can help people and families at various stages in their cancer journey. It is important not to get disheartened and give up.

Medical science has evolved by leaps and bounds, and breast cancer is completely curable by proper evidence-based treatment. India has very advanced cancer care hospitals in the private sector as well as in the public sector. There are many regional cancer centers and tertiary care hospitals that are either state or central government-owned. They are well-equipped and have all the facilities to treat all stages of breast cancer. Many medical colleges also have specialist breast surgeons as well as all the facilities for diagnosis and treatment. Sometimes, it may be difficult for the rural folk to reach these hospitals. The out-of-pocket expenses associated with cancer treatment in government hospitals are definitely less compared to that in private cancer hospitals or corporate hospitals.[3]

Before going into the specifics of cancer therapy resources, let us take a look at the healthcare structure in India. The healthcare system falls under two broad categories: Public Healthcare and Private Healthcare. The flow chart provided gives the different levels of healthcare available under each of the categories. Under public healthcare, the Central Government and the State government are responsible for the overall health needs of the entire nation. They cater to each and every citizen through the facilities, right from sub-centers and primary health centers to tertiary care centers and referral centers.

---

[3]https://www.theweek.in/news/health/2020/02/26/what-is-the-cost-of-cancer-care-in-india.html

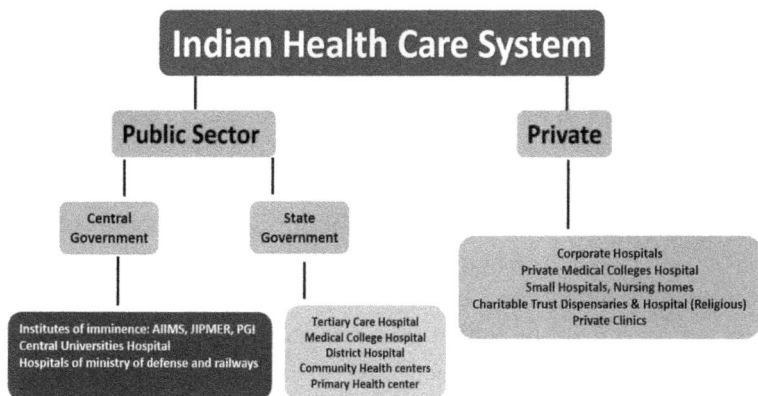

Let us first look at the resources available at government hospitals.

Therapy Resources

1. National Health Mission (NHM): Under this project, various government health workers are trained to examine and screen women for symptoms or signs of breast cancer through screening camps and primary health center (PHC) visits. Patients visiting the health sub-center or the PHC are given awareness about breast cancer and also warned about the early signs and symptoms of the same. In community health centers (CHC) and first referral units (FRU), opportunistic screening for breast cancer is done. Basically, this means you can go to the CHC/FRU and ask for a breast ultrasound to be performed.
2. Higher Centers: In higher centers, such as district hospitals, medical college hospitals, and tertiary care hospitals, all the facilities for diagnosis and management of breast cancer are present. Surgery for breast cancer is performed at the district hospital level upwards.

3. Specialized treatment options like radiation therapy, immunotherapy, and targeted therapy are available at medical colleges or tertiary care hospitals.

4. Tertiary Cancer Care Centers: They have doctors specializing in all the fields related to cancer care or oncology, such as medical oncologists, surgical oncologists, radiation therapists, and palliative care specialists.

Financial Resources

The following government schemes can help people from economically weak sections in the treatment of cancer.

1. Pradhan Mantri Jan Arogya Yojana (PM-JAY): Under this scheme, underprivileged rural families and urban workers' families can receive benefits up to rupees five lakhs per family for secondary and tertiary care hospitalizations. There is no cap on family size or age.[4]

2. Health Minister's Discretionary Grant (HMDG): For those cancer patients who have a family income below Rs. 1,25,000/- per annum, the HMDG provides financial assistance varying from Rs. 75,000/- to Rs. 1,25,000/-. This is to meet part of the expenditure on cancer treatment in government hospitals where free medical facilities are not available.[5]

3. Cancer Patient's Concession for Air Travel: Air India offers a 50 percent discount for cancer patients who are residents of India and are traveling for medical treatment.[6]

4. Health Minister's Cancer Patient Fund (HMCPF) of Rashtriya Arogya Nidhi (RAN): Patients who are below the poverty line can claim up to Rs. 2,00,000/- assistance for cancer treatment at any one of the 27 Regional Cancer

---

[4]https://pmjay.gov.in/about/pmjay
[5]https://main.mohfw.gov.in/sites/default/files/4451946500hmdgappl_1_1_0.pdf
[6]https://www.airindia.in/cancer-patients-concession.htm

Centers (RCCs) in the country. The particular RCC has the authority to process the application and dispense the fund.[7]

5. Central Government Health Scheme (CGHS): Serving and retired Central Government employees are eligible to avail of this scheme. They can get cancer treatment at approved rates from any hospital, aside from those set up under the CGHS.[8]

6. Railways: Facilities for Cancer Patients: Patients get 100 percent concession in A/C 3-tier/sleeper class, 75 percent concession in second class and A/C chair car, and 50 percent concession in A/C 2-tier and A/C first class travel. One attendant can avail 75 percent concession in A/C 3-tier/sleeper class, second class, and A/C chair car and 50 percent concession in A/C 2-tier and A/C first class.

7. Chief Minister's Relief Fund: Below poverty line patients are eligible for financial assistance from the Government of Karnataka. If the patient has already undergone the treatment, they can submit the final bills and the discharge summary.

8. Mediclaim scheme of Directorate of Health Services: This scheme is for the permanent residents of Goa. Mediclaim facility can be availed for Radiotherapy and Chemotherapy up to Rs. 5 lakhs. Treatment has to be undertaken in specific hospitals in Goa and outside Goa.[9]

9. Arogyasri Scheme of Andhra Pradesh Government: Cancer patients in AP are eligible for free treatment if their annual family income is below Rs. 5 lakhs. The AP Government has a tie-up with 150 hospitals across the state as well as in Hyderabad, Chennai, and Bangalore for rendering services under this scheme. The AP Government reimburses the

[7]https://main.mohfw.gov.in/sites/default/files/254789632565878966552HMCP F%20%281%29.pdf

[8]https://cghs.gov.in/index1.php?lang=1&level=3&sublinkid=5946&lid=3879

[9]http://www.goa.gov.in/wp-content/uploads/2020/02/Goa-Mediclaim-Scheme.pdf

costs to these hospitals. Moreover, patients receive Rs. 225/- per day for post-surgery care.

10. Cancer Suraksha Scheme by Kerala Social Security Mission: This scheme is for children suffering from cancer below 18 years of age who hail from poor families. Up to Rs. 50,000/- per child is provided by the Mission to the treating hospitals.[10]

11. Free Chemotherapy Program of the Odisha Government: All poor cancer patients residing in the state of Odisha are eligible to receive free chemotherapy. The treatment can be availed at the district hospitals in all 30 districts in the state, the Capital hospital, and the Ispat General Hospital in Rourkela.

12. Mukh Mantri Punjab Cancer Raahat Kosh Scheme: Financial assistance up to Rs. 1.5 lakhs is provided for treatment to cancer patients who are residents of Punjab. Government employees, ESI beneficiaries, ESI employees and their dependents, and patients who have health insurance or other sources of reimbursement are not eligible under this scheme.

13. State Illness Assistance Fund, Directorate of Health Services, Government of Madhya Pradesh: Any cancer patient who is domiciled in MP and is below the poverty line can avail of this treatment. The assistance provided varies from Rs 25,000/- to Rs. 2 lakhs per person.[11]

14. Free Cancer Medicines Scheme of Rajasthan Government: Drug distribution centers have been set up in government-run selected hospitals in Rajasthan. Through these counters, patients can avail themselves of 36 different types of cancer medications, which are on the essential drug list for free distribution.

---

[10]https://socialsecuritymission.gov.in/scheme_info.php?id=1
[11]https://health.mp.gov.in/en/state-illness-assistance-fund

15. Free Cancer Treatment in Government Hospitals: The West Bengal State Government has made the treatment of all types of cancers completely free in state-run hospitals and medical colleges. The service includes free medicines, radiotherapy, chemotherapy, surgical procedures, and hospital stay.

The Uttar Pradesh Government provided around Rupees 132.55/- crores from the Chief Minister's Fund to 7269 beneficiaries in the year 2020-2021 for their healthcare needs. Maximum aid was given to patients undergoing treatment for cancer, kidney diseases, and heart ailments. Apart from these schemes by the central and state governments, the people can avail themselves of many other insurance schemes.

1. Ayushman Bharat: Ayushman Bharat is a national health protection scheme that aims to provide Rs. 5 lakhs annual insurance coverage to more than 100 million poor families. It will be funded with 60 percent contribution from the central government and the remaining from the state governments. Benefits from the scheme are portable across the country.

2. Rashtriya Swasthya Bima Yojana (RSBY): This is a health insurance scheme for below poverty line families. It covers the unorganized sectors, such as construction workers, street vendors, domestic and sanitation workers, rag pickers, and rickshaw pullers.
   The beneficiaries under RSBY are entitled to hospitalization coverage up to Rs. 30,000/- per year for most diseases, including cancer care.

3. Employees State Insurance (ESI): ESI provides socio-economic protection to workers and their dependents covered under the scheme. ESI has tie-ups with recognized medical institutions to provide cashless treatment to insured people and their family members for treatments not

available in ESI institutions. This covers advanced cancer care and therapies.

4. Ex-servicemen Contributory Health Scheme: All ex-servicemen who are receiving a pension and their dependents are covered by this scheme. Cashless Medicare is availed through smart cards.

5. Private Cancer Insurance in India: A large population of people who are considered to belong to the middle-class based on their economic status is not covered by government insurance schemes. To prevent catastrophic health expenditures, these people have to depend on private health insurance plans for financial support when they fall sick.

Many private companies provide specific cancer insurance policies to cover all cancer-related healthcare expenses. The difference between regular medical insurance and a disease-specific health insurance plan, such as the cancer insurance plan, is that the former covers only the hospitalization. While the latter covers beyond in-patient hospitalization. Cancer-specific insurance plans cover these procedures. Cancer insurance policies cover most costs associated with cancer treatment, including diagnosis, biopsy and surgery, radiotherapy, chemotherapy, targeted therapies, hospitalization, and rehabilitation.

Private hospitals run by trusts and foundations play a big role in providing affordable cancer therapy for poor patients.

King George's Medical University, Lucknow:

This is a government hospital located in Lucknow, Uttar Pradesh. The Department of Endocrine Surgery is well-equipped, and we have treated numerous breast cancer patients. All the survivor stories included in this book are of women who underwent treatment in our hospital in my department.

There are many more such institutions all over the country. You can find more details on the internet.[12]

One of the major problems that cancer patients face in their treatment is the cost of accommodation and food for themselves and their accompanying family members when they have come to a different city or state for their therapy. This is a major drain on their meager finances. Many patients are not able to afford treatment or discontinue their cancer treatment midway because of the above reasons. There are many NGOs and charitable organizations that provide free or subsidized accommodation, free food, and refreshments in many of the metro cities where the cancer hospitals are located. In many of these places, patients are allowed to stay for as long as it takes to complete the cancer therapy, which is usually a long period. Food may be provided in these places, or there may be facilities that allow the patients to prepare their own food. Some of them also provide transport facilities to patients for chemotherapy or radiation therapy. More information about these NGOs and their help can be checked online at the website www.cancerassist.in.[13]

Lower middle-class people do not have private medical insurance coverage because of the high premium rates. Many NGOs also provide financial assistance to poor cancer patients. The NGOs collect donations from companies, corporate houses, and individuals and disburse them to poor patients. There are a number of such NGOs: Caring Souls Foundation, Cancer Aid and Research Foundation, Tata Trusts, Child Vikas Foundation, Sharana Breast Cancer Research and Relief Foundation, to name a few.

You can find more information online at the website www.cancerassist.in.[14] Although many cancer medications are available for free to poor patients under the many Government schemes, patients may still need to buy some patented medicines for which the generic versions are not yet made available.

[12]https://www.cancerassist.in/affordable-treatment-for-poor-patients
[13]https://www.cancerassist.in/accommodation-for-patients-and-kin
[14]https://www.cancerassist.in/financial-help-for-needy-patients

Certain drug companies, such as Pfizer and Roche, provide cancer medicines to eligible patients under patient-assist programs. Another area of distress for women suffering from breast cancer is the loss of hair following chemotherapy. NGOs provide free wigs to these women, which goes a long way toward making them feel better and restoring their confidence. Women who have undergone mastectomy are given breast implants, which again is an important service. NGOs are involved in providing counseling to cancer patients and their relatives at a very difficult time in their lives. Patients receive emotional support and motivation through these counselors, which helps them continue the treatment and not give up in despair.

I want to stress that early diagnosis and treatment of breast cancer go a long way in reducing the financial burden of the disease in the long run. A study conducted in the US reported that early detection of breast cancer through screening was generally associated with a lower cost of treatment.

The study was conducted among women aged 18 to 65 years. It found that the costs were higher for those patients diagnosed at a more advanced stage of the disease.

For stage 4 breast cancer, the chemotherapy costs were higher. The average costs provided by the insurance agents in the first year after diagnosis were as follows: For Stage 0, $60,637; for Stage I/II, $82,121; for Stage III, $129,387; for Stage IV, $134,682. Overall, the study reported that the cost of treatment was significantly higher for advanced-stage disease than that for early-stage disease. I have quoted this study to give an idea of the expenditure incurred.

However, the cost of treatment in our own country depends on the setup in which the patient is being treated. Early detection of breast cancer by routine screening leads to not only reduced morbidity and mortality but also to lower costs of treatment.[15]

---

[15]https://www.ncbi.nlm.nih.gov/pmc/articles/PMC4822976/

SURVIVOR NOTES

Bhumika is a young patient who suffered from right breast cancer. Her story exemplifies how a young girl faced cancer and fought it.

Name: Bhumika Srikant
Age: 26
Location: Rakehati, Lakhimpur

My name is Bhumika Srikant, and I am a resident of Rakehati in the district of Lakhimpur. I am a 26-year-old breast cancer warrior. I have been leading a healthy and normal life for two years now. My experience with this frightening disease revolves not only around its pain and predicament but also the financial burden cancer brings along. I am from a very humble background. My father is a daily wage earner and also the breadwinner of the family. I have witnessed the plight of many women just like me as I walked down the corridors of KGMU.

Series of diagnostic tests, an unending list of medicines, numerous injections—all these contributed to making the diagnosis of breast cancer a financial burden for a family like mine. However, I extend my gratitude to all the doctors in the Department of Endocrine Surgery at KGMU who assured me that I would be able to complete my treatment. I was informed about the various financial aids and schemes that are available for patients who hail from an underprivileged background like me.

One day, while bathing, I accidentally touched my breasts and felt a lump in my right breast. I pressed it and it was not painful. I asked my mother to check the lump. She too felt the lump but did not know what it was.

However, she realized that it was something that needed to be checked out and asked me to consult a doctor. Initially, I went to the local doctor at Lakhimpur. The lump was checked and I was advised to undergo a needle aspiration test. I never thought the lump would bring havoc to my life.

I went to the doctor once I received the report of the needle aspiration test. The reports were inconclusive, and I was referred to the Medical College Hospital at Lucknow for further evaluation immediately. It was a little terrifying. I knew that doctors usually referred their patients to the Medical College Hospital when they had serious or complicated diseases. Terribly worried, my father and I immediately left for Lucknow. I consulted a doctor at the Department of Endocrine Surgery of KGMU. Seeing my anxious face, the doctor guessed I was worried and spoke calmly and reassuringly. I underwent a biopsy of the breast mass: a slice of the breast lump was cut out and sent for testing. I was given a list of further tests that I had to undergo. The breast lump was growing slowly. I rushed back to the doctor as soon as I received the reports. The doctor, after going through the reports, spoke the most dreaded words that any woman would hear about herself.

"You have breast cancer!" I could not believe my ears. All of a sudden, I was told I had one of the most dreadful diseases humans could have—Cancer. The diagnosis of breast cancer is devastating to a woman. Breasts epitomize women. They are a symbol of womanhood, motherhood, and beauty. Where would I go now? What would happen to my life? Instead of listening to the doctor's explanation of the disease, I broke down thinking instead of the money required for the prolonged treatment. I kept muttering the same line again and again: Where would I get so much money from? My family is too poor to bear this huge cost of treatment. Hearing my concerns, the doctor assured me that the treatment would not be too exorbitant. My initial treatment was chemotherapy.

My first chemotherapy session was scheduled for October 9, 2017. I was prescribed eight sessions of chemotherapy, which took place every 14 days.

With each session, I started losing my hair, and by the end of chemotherapy, I was completely bald. My right breast was completely removed on February 12, 2018, by a surgical process and I underwent 16 radiotherapy sessions. My treatment finally concluded in May 2018. I shall be indebted to my doctors in the Department of Endocrine Surgery at KGMU.

With my inadequate knowledge of cancer and its implications and my impoverished wallet, I could never have completed my treatment without their help. The doctor acquainted me with a few organizations that helped me immensely in getting the proper treatment. Today, as I face life in a new avatar, I would request all my fellow women not to get scared.

Cancer brings in a motley of problems: physical, emotional, psychological, and of course, financial. Many like me often think of backing out of the treatment process, contemplating the costs involved. Through my story, I would like to inform you that there are many NGOs and organizations that come forward to help women from poorer backgrounds. Everyone has a right to live, whether one is born with a silver spoon or born in a slum. Do not hesitate to consult a doctor citing financial issues. Cancer is dreadful; it kills the soul more than the body.

I would like to advise every victim of cancer to have an open discussion with the doctors. KGMU has every kind of facility available to impart life to people like me.

Cancer care can be affordable. Do not lose hope.

There are many women like Bhumika who are utterly crushed on hearing the diagnosis of cancer. If they hail from a poor or underprivileged background, the one dominating thought looming in their minds is the cost of treatment. Treatment of advanced breast cancer is complicated, prolonged, and expensive. Many times, patients leave the treatment midway for financial reasons or opt for other less expensive 'pathies.'

Any big expense can plunge them into irretrievable and lifelong debt. They develop a sense of fatality and have the attitude of 'what will be, will be.' They make up their minds to face the disease with fortitude rather than bring financial disaster to the family. It is imperative that these patients be educated about these resources and how they can avail themselves of their help.

Beena suffered from carcinoma left breast. Her tumor was triple negative. She did not have any children. She underwent a total mastectomy followed by chemotherapy and loco-regional radiation in 2017.

Name: Beena Mishra
Age: Undisclosed
Location: Undisclosed

Life is never a bed of roses. We all face setbacks and severe challenges that we need to overcome in life. And during the course of our life, we often come across God in the disguise of humans. They hold us up and help to overcome the hurdles. They stand by our side to show us the dazzling ray of hope at the end of the tunnel.

My name is Beena Mishra. I am a woman: a daughter, raised with immense love and care, a caring daughter-in-law, a doting wife, and a loving aunt. And these days, a new tag defines me in this mortal world. I am a breast cancer survivor.

Yes! I have survived one of the most dreadful diseases of human life. Having been through the long haul of chemotherapy and radiation therapy and experienced the overpowering burden of never-ending medicines and injections, I could fathom how a disease, a mishap, could rebuild my core strength. On April 2, 2016, while taking a shower, I noticed a slight difference in my left breast. It felt harder than usual, and I could discern a nodule and the nipple felt a little caved-in.

A slight hardening of the breasts was a normal phenomenon, and it often happened during one of the phases of the menstrual cycle. However, I had never seen my nipples retracted before. A little concerned, I informed my husband. Unaware of the gravity of the situation, we both decided to go to a doctor.

We went to a private hospital in Faizabad and consulted a lady doctor. She made me sit and lie down in different postures and examined my breast. I was unsure when asked how long I had had the nodule. The doctor wanted me to get an ultrasound scan done first. She said that a retracted nipple was not a good sign and I would eventually need to undergo a biopsy to rule out cancer. Biopsy was related to cancer. My eyes were now glazed with fear. Seeing the fear on my face the doctor said, "Mrs. Mishra! Don't panic. Your treatment is possible. You'll be cured. You get the test done and meet me with the reports. Lucknow Medical College has all the facilities available... So don't think of cancer right now. We have to first confirm the cause and then think of the remedies."

Crying was not going to solve anything. Just like any other person would under these circumstances, I felt an unfathomable fear sink in. I got the breast ultrasound done, but the report did not clearly identify the cause of the lump. So, I was referred to Lucknow for a specialist consultation. While I pen down my thoughts today, I realize how prudent this doctor was. She did not waste any time in getting me to the specialists, thereby ensuring that the disease did not progress further. The school I was working in was closing down for the summer vacation on May 17. Not wishing to delay the diagnosis, I decided to go to Lucknow on the very next day, that is, May 18. I had to go alone as my husband had other responsibilities.

My husband came to drop me at the bus stop. I put on a brave face as I bid him goodbye. However, as the bus rushed on the highway, tears welled up in my eyes. I could no longer hold in my emotions. I failed to understand what my fault could be. I wanted to bear a child. I wanted to enjoy the bliss of motherhood. And instead of giving life to my womb, God had gifted me this dreadful disease.

I recalled the doctor's positive words, but it is human nature to anticipate the worst. My father was waiting for me at the other end and I got down and held him tight. I never realized how much I cried on his shoulder that day. All my father could do was take me home.

As I crossed the threshold, my mother rushed to me and hugged me tightly. "Why didn't you come here earlier? Why didn't you tell me before? I would have taken you to the best of the doctors…" My mother probably said a hundred other things that day. Some I heard, some were just lost in the wind.

The next morning, my younger brother scheduled an appointment at a private hospital. My mother and brother accompanied me. After going through all my reports, the doctor examined my breasts. There was fear and a lot of other emotions going through my mind. I was advised to do an FNAC test of the lump. The test was painful: a pinching pain that left a sore feeling on the breast. When the reports were ready, the doctor confirmed the presence of a tumor. The doctor wanted a biopsy to be done. After some discussion, the family decided it was best for me to go to KGMU for the biopsy and further treatment as there were experienced consultants there.

When we reached the KGMU old building the next day, I found it crowded with patients as well as doctors, junior doctors, and other hospital staff, and we were confused. I had to ask an employee who informed me that the endocrine surgery department took care of breast problems. We reached the place, and there again, the long wait started. The doctor at the endocrine surgery department looked at my reports and again checked my breasts. He too said I had to undergo a biopsy and scheduled my biopsy for the next day. The reports would take 10 to 12 days to be ready and the treatment could be started only then. I was advised to undergo the complete treatment and not leave halfway. I was struggling with the uncertainty about my future. The whole family was worried about me. I was not thinking right, and nothing or no one could console me. However, my husband was already burdened with filial responsibilities.

How could I pressurize him? I spoke to him over the phone and he perhaps understood my state of mind. He promised to be by my side forever. Somewhere, his reassuring words shored up my confidence, and it was then that I decided I would completely overcome every bit of this disease. I had to. For the loving family I had (still have), I had to fight this battle with cancer and claim victory over it.

The next day, the biopsy was done and the sample submitted to the pathology department. And then the wait began.

The days seemed longer than usual. Those 10 days were probably the longest days of my life. I wanted the reports to come early so that the treatment could be started. When the report finally arrived, the diagnosis of cancer was confirmed. I was advised first to undergo surgery with complete removal of the breast. The doctor's words robbed us of our senses. Removing a breast from a woman's body? We could not understand. We blinked at each other, not knowing what to do next.

There were some more tests that were necessary before proceeding with the operation. My operation was scheduled for a Monday. The doctor pronounced everything in such a soothing manner as if he was talking about shopping at Lucknow. It was simple for him, probably because, as a doctor, his goal was to cure his patients at any cost. No apprehension, no prejudices, and no judgments. He just saw me as a patient fighting a dreadful disease and wanted to heal my problem.

Was it the same for us? Of course, not! Breast removal (mastectomy) was beyond our understanding and acceptance. I had to repeat all the painful details to my husband over the phone. After all, he was my life partner. He did have a say in my treatment. Hearing my tearful and trembling voice, he decided to come over and asked me to be patient for a little while more. Within two to three hours, my husband settled his other responsibilities and came to me. My joy knew no bounds. He consoled me and advised me to go for the operation. "We need you to be completely cured and nothing else. Beauty will come and go.

Your life matters the most. We are all with you." He assured me. His presence by my side and his words made me stronger and more determined to win over the disease. More than anything physical, it was emotional torture for a middle-aged woman like me. My younger brother's wife was pregnant. She herself was not keeping very well, but she continually looked out for everyone at home. Running here and there, she was consoling the family members and convincing them that everything would be alright. She took care of everyone at home, persuading them to eat. We were going about our days mechanically, running between different doctors and collecting reports. It probably took ten days or a week for me to get all my tests done. And now, I was all set to start with the treatment procedures.

My operation was scheduled for June 22, 2016, so I was admitted a day before. My husband and I kept talking about the good times in our lives. We relived our past memories. All through my married life, I had seen my husband as a strong man who could carry out every responsibility without ever demonstrating any worry or fear.

The same night, I also called up the principal of the school where I worked to inform her about all the developments. The school was scheduled to reopen on June 25, and it was necessary to keep her in the loop. I requested her to grant me leave from my school duties. I was overwhelmed by her response. She was so encouraging and optimistic about my treatment. A big burden of responsibility was taken off my shoulders. The new dawn was different. I woke up with an optimistic outlook. Soon, I was called for the operation. My husband and I went and sat in the waiting hall near the operation theatre. Just as my name was called, my brother and parents came in. As I was moved inside the operation theatre (OT), I had just one thought—*Hope to see my family soon*. Big room, gigantic machines, and doctors and nurses all garbed in their OT aprons. All the specialists were inside the OT. Masked and gloved, they all set to operate on me. The last thing I remember is someone placing the anesthesia mask over my face and then, everything was black. I remembered nothing after that. I was in the emergency ward when I regained consciousness.

As soon as the effects of the anesthesia wore off, I started feeling the real pain of the operation. I could see the pity in everyone's eyes. I pitied myself too. Did I just lose my womanhood?

Visiting time was over. All the other relatives left while my husband and mother remained by my side. My mother was not well, but still, she chose to be with me. They both stood like pillars of strength. The night waned out with me lying still on the bed. A physiotherapist came in and taught me three to four exercises, which I followed despite the unbearable pain.

Initially, I had very severe pain in the back. Almost everyone in the family came to see me. They applauded my courage and asked me to hold aloft this confidence. My father dropped in every single day, both in the morning and in the evening.

Seeing so many different kinds of people in the hospital and hearing their stories, I realized that none of us was trouble-free. We all had our share of joy and sorrow.

We encouraged each other to get well soon. We were building a support system for each other. I was discharged on the seventh day, which happened to be my birthday as well. To welcome me, the family had cooked a lot of dishes at home. Everyone enjoyed the food and went to bed. However, I could not rest. The pain persisted and it was unbearable in the beginning. I cried on my mother's lap more from the pain of losing a part of my body than from the pain of the surgery. The physical pain was manageable to a large extent with the pain medications prescribed to me. My husband continued to stand by me like an emotional pillar, consoling me to be strong. He diligently ensured that I took all the medicines. The idea is usually ingrained in a girl child during her growing years that her ultimate role in life would be that of a wife and mother.

She is brought up with the mindset of taking care of her family, seeing to her filial duties, performing her marital roles, and bearing children. While that year, all the others at our home had taken over my duties and were trying to do their bit. I went for a review to KGMU on the 12th day, and after checking the wound, suture removal was done.

I was advised that I might experience some irregularity or cessation of the menstrual cycle owing to cancer therapy. I thought, breast gone, periods gone, what was the purpose of me being a woman? After three weeks, I returned to the hospital with my biopsy report for further treatment. The chemo medicines were prescribed and I was also given detailed information about the side effects of chemotherapy. Vomiting, fatigue, mouth ulcers, loose bowel, and hair loss seemed to be the common ones. I had one question: Can I continue to work? The answer: I could, provided I was careful about cleanliness. I was told to avoid crowded places and eat only home-cooked food. I was administered the first chemo dose on July 18. The session ran for six hours, from 5 p.m. to 11 p.m., and then I was allowed to come back home. I started experiencing discomfort the next morning. I felt queasy in the stomach; there was mild nagging pain and occasional cramping in the abdomen.

I started vomiting. Everyone in the house was ready to get me anything I wished to eat; however, I did not know what to eat. My taste buds seemed to be dead.

Gradually, a week passed by. I was frail, unable to even walk. My mouth was filled with painful ulcers. I went to KGMU for a check-up and I was administered an immunity-building injection. I went back to my home after three months. Everyone was eagerly waiting to meet me. My mother-in-law and my sister-in-law and her kids all loved me very much. We all spent the night speaking about every odd thing under the sky. None of us slept that night. The next morning, I was all set to join the school. Some of my colleagues were on the bus. They all enquired about my health. I was overwhelmed by so much love surrounding me.

The director of the institute where I worked blessed me to get cured completely and also approved my application for leave whenever I had chemo sessions. The help, support, and blessings I received were akin to a life-saving armor. When I started losing my hair, my husband chopped off all the tangled tufts of hair with a pair of scissors. I even got my periods after the first session of chemotherapy.

I did not have a child yet; I was indeed worried about that as well. When I shared my concerns with the doctors in the Department of Endocrine Surgery, I was advised a few tests and procedures in case I got my periods. Preserving my ova was another option open to me. They had even discussed my case with an experienced doctor at another hospital. Once I got cured, I could use the preserved ova myself or opt for surrogacy. I was certainly cautioned about the expenses involved. We looked into the possibility of preserving my ova at the other hospital. I underwent a lot of tests. The specialists there discussed my issues and told me that the treatment would cost around eight to ten lakh rupees. As I was undergoing chemotherapy, there was no guarantee that my ova were viable enough. After hearing about the chances of preserving a healthy ovum, we decided not to pursue the option any further.

By December 1, all six sessions of chemotherapy were over. Except for one session, my blood profile was normal throughout the process. During the third session of my chemo, my sister-in-law gave birth to a son. I was so elated that as soon as my chemo was over, I rushed to the hospital to meet the newborn and the mother. I played with the baby. Everyone was happy in the house. Nobody realized how swiftly we moved through 21 days. It was Navratri once my fourth chemo was over. Somehow, I was able to help my mother in all the preparations from the third day onwards. My hair gradually started growing back after the fifth chemo. Another 21 days went by, and by December, I had received my sixth chemo session too.

Memories are peculiar.

Some memories make us cry and some make us prance with joy, while a few memories remain alive always and serve to make us believe in our inherent strength. I have kept all those fallen strands of hair to date. They still smell of oils and shampoo. Some may find it curious. But, when I see them, I realize what I could overcome. The next course of action was radiotherapy. My first radiotherapy session was scheduled for January 26. My course of treatment seemed unending. Even though we had a normal lifestyle, my treatment costs were sky-rocketing.

I forced my husband to look out for a new job. I was stronger than before, and I could manage on my own for the radiotherapy sessions.

Radiotherapy was scheduled for every day of the week except for Saturdays and Sundays. My father and my brother had their own businesses to take care of. *Bahadur Bhaiya* stepped in to take care of me during my radiotherapy sessions. He used to help my father in the construction work. He accompanied me during the 16 sessions and took care of all the hospital formalities.

As I sit and recollect my memories, I find so many blessings I was bestowed with. God does not come in his own avatar maybe. But he does send his blessings through such kind souls. I shall always be indebted to *Bahadur Bhaiya*. I met my doctor once the treatment was over. He advised me to come every three months for a review check-up to ensure that all was fine.

Nowadays, my review happens once in six months. All my reports are normal and I no longer have any health issues. I have recovered completely and am leading a normal and healthy life like before. This new life came to me as a blessing and I wish to direct it toward some noble work. My only aim is to help all those people suffering from such a dreadful disease. I am thoroughly indebted to all the doctors, junior doctors, nursing staff, hospital staff, ward boys, and helpers, and everyone else as well, who played a crucial role in my treatment process. My parents stood beside me through all the difficult circumstances and lent me physical, emotional, and financial support.

'Thanks' will be too small a word for my mother-in-law, sister-in-law and her husband, co-sister, and the kids who kept in touch regularly by phone and encouraged me to complete the treatment. They all were like a constant ray of hope.

I do not know how to thank my younger brother, his wife, and her sister, who remained with us for six months and took immense care of me and my family. Lots of love and blessings to my daughter, who was not born out of my womb but took care of me like she would her own mother, undeterred by her duties.

She never let me realize that I am childless. My blessings are always with you. I wish all your dreams come true. On the same note, I thank the whole society of JBNSS, my Director Madam, Principal, Vice-Principal, Coordinator Madam, my colleagues, assistants, and the school children. Their undying support, love, and blessings helped me hold my confidence. And not to forget, I shall remain grateful to *Bahadur Bhaiya* for all the timely help.

I am a common woman—a middle-class working lady who could never have conceived such an atrocious design of destiny. As I come out of my cancer battlefield, I realize the sheer significance of taking care of one's health. I write this memoir not only to thank my doctors but to raise awareness about breast cancer.

A woman's breast is not just a sign of her beauty and a mode to feed her children. It is complex and it requires attention. A woman remains the backbone of a family. While we endeavor to nourish others, we must look after ourselves as well. My sincere advice to all new patients is not to lose hope and be courageous during the treatment.

Do not get overwhelmed with all that cancer therapy entails.
Accept help when needed.

Beena narrates the whole experience of her fight with cancer. As a woman, there is a lot to face when you are suddenly diagnosed to have breast cancer.

In addition to facing drastic changes, such as mastectomy and losing all her hair, the family had to meet the costs involved as well for targeted immunotherapy. Luckily, she had the support of her family. Her relatives stepped up to give the necessary funds. While the majority of chemotherapy drugs can be accessed for free at Public Hospitals, targeted innovative therapies are still not free.

In our country, it is a reality that still many of the poorer patients do not seek treatment for breast cancer fearing the costs involved. The financial burden of cancer therapy is very high for those below the poverty limit or in underprivileged households.

Empowering women and communities by increasing awareness of the benefits of early diagnosis can go a long way in overcoming this hesitancy. Another step that would improve treatment rates in breast cancer therapy is making people aware of the numerous resources that they can avail themselves of with regard to government schemes, insurance policies, funding, hospitals that offer subsidized treatment, accommodation and food, and counseling and support. Once a diagnosis of breast cancer is made, how do you decide where to go for the treatment? It is important to make the right choices here. Let us see how to opt for scientifically proven treatment methods in the next chapter.

4

PLANNING CANCER THERAPY: THE BEST WAY FORWARD

It is all about choosing the right treatment

Cancer is a complex disease that includes a series of gene–environment interactions in a progressive process that requires the malfunction of DNA repair, apoptosis, and immunological functions. A doctor, from day one of his professional life, takes the pledge to treat the illnesses of patients with utmost care and sincerity. The objective of cancer therapy is to cure cancer and restore the ability to live a normal life. Any cancer therapy can be used as the first line of defense; nevertheless, surgery is the most frequent initial cancer treatment for the most common malignancies. Some cancers are very susceptible to radiation therapy or chemotherapy; in such a case, you may receive one of these therapies as your primary treatment. Adjuvant therapy is the measure taken to kill any cancer cells that remain after the first 'surgery' treatment.

This lowers the likelihood of recurrence. Adjuvant therapies include chemotherapy, radiation therapy, and hormone therapy. When the cancer is in advanced stages and a cure is not likely, the emphasis is on stabilizing the patient, controlling the symptoms, and prolonging life.

In very advanced stages of the disease, the focus shifts to palliation of symptoms and keeping the patient as happy and comfortable as possible, and later, end-of-life care as required.

It is important to note that cancer can be cured in the early stages with timely adequate treatment. Breast cancer begins in the tissues of the breast. Breast cancer, like other malignancies, has the ability to enter and expand into the tissues that surround the breast. It can also spread to other regions of the body, resulting in the formation of additional tumors, a process known as metastasis. Treatment of breast cancer is planned after adequate investigation. Initial investigations are triple tests that include detailed clinical history and examination, imaging, and a core biopsy of the lump. Of all diagnostic investigations, the most important one is the core biopsy. Biopsy provides a lot of information like the type of cancer and which treatment will be better for the patient. After this diagnostic investigation, the patient is asked to undergo further investigations, which give us information about the cancer stage. The staging of breast cancer tells us whether the tumor is restricted to only the breast or has spread beyond the breast to the axilla or to other organs of the body. Treatment protocols are different for different stages of breast cancer. The treatment is personalized and depends upon the type of cancer, stage and grade, and presence of metastases.

Stage 1 breast cancer is when the tumor is limited to the breast and is less than two centimeters in size. If cancer is affecting the breast as well as the axilla and seems to be operable, then it is stage 2. Stage 3 cancer is when it is large or advanced and has spread to the chest wall or skin of the breast. When cancer has spread to other organs of the body, it is stage 4. With modern-day treatment, cancer is a curable disease. It is no more a disease that summons death.

There are numerous instances where I have witnessed breast cancer patients who, on becoming aware of their symptoms, sought medical help on time and were completely cured. But the notion of cancer and the associated misinformation has led people to seek alternative measures. Delaying or refusing 'evidence-based' conventional cancer therapy (CCT) in favor of alternative medicine might have major bad consequences for cancer patients' survival.

However, due to data paucity or patient reluctance to reveal nonmedical therapy to their doctors, there is minimal study analyzing the usage and effectiveness of alternative medicine. People opt for alternative medicine because of their unawareness and the taboos that endorse their minds. Patients start searching the internet and social media for information. One may come across many scientific-sounding articles or videos of "medical experts," which may offer new hope and cure and describe the treatments as "all natural" without any unpleasant or serious side effects. These sites even include testimonials from patients or their family members, who describe miraculous results. This information may sound too good to be true, but they are disastrous to the patients as it drags them away from scientifically proven evidence-based medicine to an unknown, unpredictable territory. This misinformation not only results in suffering for the cancer patients themselves, but also for the entire family.

In a study by Skylar B Johnson et al. on the 'Use of Alternative Medicine for Cancer and its impact on Survival,' 281 individuals with non-metastatic breast, prostate, lung, or colorectal cancer were reported to have opted for alternative medical therapies for anticancer treatment after failing to respond to traditional cancer treatment, which included chemotherapy, radiation, surgery, and hormone therapy[16]. It was found that alternative medicine usage was independently related to a higher risk of mortality compared to conventional cancer treatment.

---

[16]jnci: Journal of the National Cancer Institute, Volume 110, Issue 1, January 2018, Pages 121–124, https://doi.org/10.1093/jnci/djx145

For breast cancer, women who had alternative medicine as their first therapy without cancer treatment had a five-fold greater risk of mortality. In Western nations, the average prevalence of alternative medicine use among cancer patients is 40 percent. An article exploring the use of alternative medicine in Bangladesh concludes that seeking medical help other than the orthodox available treatment leads to the delayed presentation by breast cancer patients.[17]

Alternative medicine's idea, practice, kind, and technique of application vary greatly across ethnic groups residing in different areas of the nation, depending on their culture, living standards, economic status, religious beliefs, and educational level. Homeopathy, Unani, and Ayurvedic systems are practiced in India and Bangladesh. Many cancer patients use homeopathy in cancer treatment with the perception that it will boost their bodies' ability to fight cancer, enhance immunity, improve physical and mental well-being, and relieve pain caused by cancer or conventional therapies. These alternative therapies may help in relieving the pain and providing treatment satisfaction in patients with advanced terminal cancer. The major reasons for the initial use of alternative medicine in the treatment of breast cancer are probably low per capita income, a low literacy rate, high diagnostic and treatment costs, and easy access to alternative medicine. Alternative medicine can be used in a complementary role in advanced-stage patients but should never be used as the first or initial option. Alternative therapies have always resulted in disease progression and early mortality when used as a first-line option for treating breast cancer.

A study of breast cancer patients, published in the World Journal of Surgery in 2012, looked at 185 women in the Northern Alberta Health Region who declined evidence-based treatment, and concluded that patients who declined primary standard treatment had significantly worse survival than those who received standard treatments.

---

[17]https://cms.galenos.com.tr/Uploads/Article_42040/ejbh-14-166-En.pdf

There was no evidence to support that using alternative medicine as the primary cancer treatment option helped these patients.[18] One has to understand that alternative medicine is sometimes quite expensive with high charges per sitting and has a huge impact financially on the family. One of the wrongly held beliefs is that by doing a biopsy or with a touch of metal, cancer spreads faster. It is a piece of totally false information, and fine-needle aspiration cytology (FNAC) or core biopsy, in which a core of tissue is removed by a specialized needle, is totally safe.

The information obtained through FNAC or biopsy is vital for the oncologist to plan the correct treatment for the patient. The core of tissue taken in the biopsy not only confirms the presence of cancer but also tells the type of cancer by studying the cells involved; this allows the oncologist to predict the behavior of the cancer. A biopsy also helps in deciding which cancer drugs (chemotherapy) will be more effective and if surgery is indicated.

In my 25 years of experience with breast cancer treatment, I have come across so many patients with initial stage cancer, some from very educated backgrounds, who left us either during the initial stages of the treatment or during the middle of the treatment and later, after six to nine months, and when cancer has advanced or become metastatic, came back realizing their mistake. One has to understand what happens when you stop receiving treatment for breast cancer.

A simple lump in the breast will gradually increase in size and eventually become adherent to the surrounding structures in the breast; it can get fixed to the chest wall and can involve the overlying skin. As the tumor progresses, it can become softened in some places and burst through the skin. This progression depends upon the type and grade of cancer. The alternative medicine practitioners play with the psychology of the patient and their relatives. They explain this progression in their way.

---

[18]https://www.ncbi.nlm.nih.gov/pmc/articles/PMC3438047/

They explain that the treatment is working, and the lump that was deep-seated initially is becoming more obvious, and once it bursts, they will say that the dirty blood and cancer worms are getting drained out from the wound through the ulcer. Sometimes social media posts may hold appeal because they align with people's pre-existing, deeply held false beliefs. We must confront the problem head-on by working with our patients, alerting them to the kind of misinformation they may face, and providing them with proper sources of information to explore. According to a study published in the Journal of the National Cancer Institute in July 2021, one-third of the most widely viewed cancer treatment articles on social media provide inaccurate information[19].

Misinformation can lead to 'harmful inaction'; this, in turn, can result in delay or refusal of medical attention for treatable/curable conditions, economic harm, and harmful interactions.

- Harmful inaction: may result in delaying or refusing medical treatment for treatable/curable diseases, 31 percent.
- Economic damage: out-of-pocket expenditures connected with treatment/travel, 27.7 percent.
- Harmful action: possibly harmful consequences of the indicated test/treatment, 17 percent.
- Harmful interactions: known/unknown medical interactions with curative therapies, 6.2 percent.

More than three-quarters of the articles that included misinformation (76.9%; n = 50 of 65) contained detrimental material. Furthermore, most of the information cautioned that evidence-based therapies like chemotherapy are inefficient or hazardous and that traditional medicine should not be believed[20]

[19]https://academic.oup.com/jnci/advance-article-abstract/doi/10.1093/jnci/djab141/6323231?redirectedFrom=fulltext
[20]https://www.healio.com/news/hematology-oncology/20210825/inaccurate-harmful-cancer-information-prevalent-on-social-media

The 'IDIOT syndrome' (Internet-Derived Information Obstructing Treatment) is said to occur when people blindly trust all the medical information available online and stop their treatment abruptly without consulting their doctor.

To reduce the effect of harmful social media misinformation, we are required to work on the following several components:

- Patient education and cancer awareness is the most important component of this. This can be done through social media.
- We need to research and identify individuals at risk for encountering and believing misinformation, and then interventions can be done at the proper time that might help modify their behavior.
- Identification of predictors of misinformation and alert patients to this potential harm.
- Addressing social media misinformation at the policy level.

This is especially true on social media, where incorrect information travels far more quickly and widely than fact-checked information. Misinformation on cancer treatment is a public health concern and must be addressed immediately because it obstructs the delivery of evidence-based care, harms patient-physician relationships, and increases the risk of mortality. Because patients rely on social media for health information, combating misinformation should be one of the top priorities for public health officials.

Another issue prevalent in India is the superstitious faith in pseudo messiahs claiming to cure diseases. So, many patients, instead of receiving proper medical guidance, will delay and lose their scope of getting better by performing various faith-based rites and rituals promoted by these false healers. A similar incident was covered by the National News Media when a 'baba' claimed to cure cancer with a 'stone.' So how do we handle this? We need proper treatment in order to get well, especially if the disease is breast cancer, which is curable when treated timely with advances in medical science.

SURVIVOR NOTES

Anita is also a young survivor of right breast cancer. Her story too highlights how she fought the disease and gives important pointers to other breast cancer patients.

Name: Anita Chaudhary
Age: 32
Location: Lucknow

I am Anita Chaudhary, and I am 32 years old. I am married and have two children, a daughter aged eight years and a son who is five years old, and I live in Lucknow. My husband, Niraj Chaudhary, is a bank employee. I live in a joint family with my husband's parents and his younger brother's family. I am a housewife and my days start and end while looking after my home and family. We are a close-knit family and share all our joys and sorrows. The walls of our house are always resounding with joy and laughter. Being the "*badi bahu*" or the elder daughter-in-law, I have a lot of responsibilities in running the household. I take care of all the members of my family and see to their every need. My hands are always full with some work or the other. My parents live in a village close to Lucknow, and I visit them once in three or four months. I always stay for a few days and get absolutely pampered by the entire extended family there. It becomes a time for me to rest and rejuvenate, and I tend to catch up with all the family gossip.

Life was moving along on an even keel when all of a sudden, everything turned upside down. That fateful day of April 15, 2019, shall always stay in my memory. I discovered two lumps in my right breast. I had very little knowledge about breast lumps but recalled my sister-in-law telling me something about it when I had last visited my hometown.

She mentioned that my "*Maasi*" or maternal aunt was being treated for a breast swelling that she had neglected in the early stages. I called up my sister-in-law that evening after completing all my house chores, and she suggested I visit a homeopathic doctor who had treated one of her relatives. She assured me that after taking the homeo medicines, her relative had been completely cured, and the breast lump had disappeared. As per her advice, I visited the homeopathic clinic in Lucknow and started taking the medicines prescribed. However, as the days went by, I noticed that one of the lumps had disappeared, but the other seemed to have grown bigger and more prominent now. I now began to worry and called up my sister-in-law again.

She immediately wanted to know how I was faring and if the homeopathic treatment had helped. I said, "Forget the homeo treatment. Tell me what happened to your *Maasi*."

There was complete silence at the other end. My sister-in-law then revealed that her *Maasi* had delayed treatment for her swelling, which was later diagnosed as breast cancer. She had 4th-stage cancer now that had spread to other areas, and presently, she was living in Kanpur with her elder son for treatment in the city.

I started to panic now. I immediately spoke about this to my mother-in-law and my husband. My mother-in-law calmed me down and encouraged me to think positively. She took me to a nearby gynecologist the same evening for a consultation. The date was May 6, 2019, about three weeks since I had discovered the breast lumps. After examining me, the doctor instructed me to undergo a mammography test. I had mammography the very next day. After going through the mammogram report the next evening, the doctor referred me to King George's Medical University. We consulted in the endocrine surgery department. The doctor carefully listened to my story, examined me, and went through the mammogram report as well. Then I heard the words I had been dreading: I had breast cancer. Both my husband and I braced ourselves for the next step. The doctor gave us hope and courage and outlined the treatment plan.

I underwent some blood tests, ultrasound scanning, FNAC of axillary node, and core biopsy of the lump. After the test results were ready, my surgery was first planned. I underwent surgery on May 31, 2019. My post-operative recovery was uneventful, but within a month, the next round of treatment began.

Cancer is, as they say, an aggressive illness, and thus the treatment is aggressive too. Prolonged treatment is prescribed, which includes surgery, chemotherapy, and radiation therapy. I had eight cycles of chemotherapy, which commenced on June 29, 2019, and ended on October 5, 2019. It was definitely a difficult time for me. I experienced a lot of side effects like severe nausea and vomiting after each session of chemotherapy. I had lost my appetite completely and had also developed ulcers in my mouth.

My mother came over to Lucknow and stayed with me for nearly six months after my operation. She and my mother-in-law took great pains to prepare tasty and easily digestible food for me. Everyone in the family tried to help me in some or the other way. My brother-in-law always brought back new issues of magazines for me to read whenever he went out. They always tried to cheer me up and did not allow me to feel bogged down at any time. Despite all their efforts, I lost a lot of weight during this period. The presence of our loved ones makes a whole lot of difference at difficult times in our lives. I was able to mentally relax at this time because of my mother's presence. She took over many of my duties, especially looking after both my children.

I also had the support of the doctors and all the staff from the endocrine surgery department of KGMU. I was in touch with them constantly throughout my chemotherapy period, and they were always available to give me support, encouragement, and advice whenever I needed it. My doctors and family members thoroughly supervised my well-being. Such a strong support system plays a huge role in a person's recovery. I insist every patient not hesitate while asking for help. Do not hesitate to accept help. The battle is difficult, and you need all the support you can get. I underwent some more tests at the end of the chemotherapy sessions.

In December, when my children had their winter break, I visited my hometown for a couple of weeks. I went along with my children, and the ambiance around was so happy that we all could forget the dread of cancer. We could spend some happy days with all our relatives. It was a memorable time for us, except for one sad news we received just a day before the children and I returned to Lucknow. We heard that my *Maasi*, who was being treated for Stage 4 breast cancer, passed away. The news saddened me terribly, but I realized the importance of seeking early and scientifically proven treatment for a breast lump. On January 8, 2020, my radiotherapy sessions started. I approached the New Year with a refreshing hope in my heart. I had come a long way in this battle against breast cancer, and I decided not to back out now. I underwent 16 sessions of radiotherapy, with the final one scheduled on January 28, 2020. I will always be grateful that I could get treatment at a premier institution like KGMU. It is a wonderful hospital with all the required medical, surgical, and diagnostic services under one roof.

I will never forget the care and concern shown by the doctors and all the staff who work in the endocrine surgery department. I believe that it is one of the most exemplary medical departments in the institute. I want to especially mention the doctor who treated me.

I believe he gave me a new life. I shall always be grateful for his crucial role in strengthening my vigor to fight cancer. He indeed helped me in maintaining my emotional and mental balance. By the grace of God, I am healthy now. My doctors have said that I am cancer-free. Of course, I need regular follow-up, which is very crucial. Regular follow-up is useful in the early detection of recurrence, if any. To all those reading my story, I want to stress two points. Do not ever neglect a breast lump. It may not be serious, but always get it confirmed by an experienced doctor.

Moreover, women should be aware of their family history. If your siblings, mother, or mother's siblings have breast cancer, you need to go for a regular check-up.

Breast cancer does run in the family. There is a genetic connection.

I recall Swami Vivekananda's motto: Nar Seva Narayan Seva! He believed serving man is akin to serving God. The doctors and the staff at KGMU are living examples of this. I thank them from the bottom of my heart.

Know your family history. Do not ever neglect a breast lump.

Anita's experience brings home the importance of being aware of one's family history and seeking scientifically proven treatment methods at the earliest. In spite of having a close family member already diagnosed with breast cancer, Anita's relatives pointed her to alternative medicine when she presented with a lump in her breast. Sometimes, seeking these alternative therapies leads to a delay in starting proven cancer therapy. This delay can prove extremely costly when cancer that was in Stage 1 or 2 spreads and reaches Stage 4. The chances of a cure and survival are lower when you reach the advanced stages. The pain from the disease is greater and the treatment is more expensive too.

How is Breast Cancer Treated?
Breast cancer treatment involves the following:

1. Surgery: An operation where cancer from the breast is removed. It may be total removal of the breast or partial removal of the breast, which is known as conservative breast surgery. In conservative breast surgery, the remaining breast tissue can be reconstructed with volume displacement or replacement. Breast preserving operations are totally safe in terms of disease recurrence. During surgery for breast cancer, the axillary lymph nodes are addressed in all patients. This is because breast cancer first spreads to the axillary lymph nodes before disseminating to other places in the body. Nowadays, there are various modifications to axillary surgery, and it has to be individualized for each patient.

2. Chemotherapy: These are special medicines used to treat cancer and kill or stabilize the cancer cells.
3. Hormonal therapy. It blocks the cancer cells from getting the hormones that they require to grow.
4. Biological therapy or targeted therapy.
5. Radiation therapy.

The treatment of breast cancer depends on the stage of the disease. Broadly, treatment can be classified into two types: local treatment and systemic treatment. In the initial stages of cancer or stage 1 and stage 2 cancer, treatment is surgery followed by systemic treatment.

In advanced cancers, there is always the fear that cancer will spread to distant organs; therefore, for all these patients, chemotherapy is given initially with the aim of downstaging the tumor size, making it more manageable, and simultaneously, it also works on the cancer cells in the blood circulation.

In metastatic tumors, there is no role for local treatment because cancer has already spread into the different organs of the body, and by treating cancer locally alone, the patient will not be benefited. So, in summary, in the initial stages, surgery is the first treatment followed by chemotherapy and radiation, while in advanced tumors, chemotherapy is the first treatment followed by surgery and radiation. Targeted chemotherapy is also available nowadays, but who will benefit from targeted therapy depends on the results of the core biopsy.

Which Course of Treatment is the Best for Breast Cancer?

Most patients require a combination of three treatment modalities: surgery, chemotherapy, and radiation. Which treatment should be first and which one second depends upon factors like patient age, stage of disease, menopausal status, and core biopsy results. Breast cancer treatment is highly individualized now, and there is no single treatment pattern that can be called the best.

How Long is the Treatment Duration of Breast Cancer?

Treatment for breast cancer usually lasts three to eight months. A minimum of six to eight months is usually necessary for advanced-stage cancers.

Breakdown of the Treatment Duration:

From the onset of the first symptom until the initial consultation, there is a time delay. The treatment duration is as follows:
1. Time spent during investigations for diagnostic purposes.
2. Surgical procedures (includes recovery and interval to other treatment): four to six weeks.
3. Chemotherapy is administered once every three weeks for six sessions. The whole cycle takes around 18 weeks to complete. Interval of four weeks before the next treatment.
4. Six weeks of radiotherapy (commonest scenario).

Total amount of time taken usually is in between: 4-6 weeks + 18 weeks + 4 weeks + 6 weeks = 34 weeks = 8 months

Treatment Delays

Because primary prevention of breast cancer is currently unavailable, efforts to increase early identification remain the primary emphasis in the battle against the disease. Minimizing delays in the detection, diagnosis, and treatment of breast cancer is critical. Longer wait periods between the diagnosis and start of treatment have been linked to stage advancement, disease worsening, and treatment problems. Delay can be divided into two categories: patient delay and system delay. Patient delay refers to a patient's failure to seek medical help after self-discovering a possible breast cancer symptom, and system delay refers to the time it takes for patients to get appointments, schedule diagnostic testing, receive a final diagnosis, and begin treatment.

Both of these factors may result in a worse prognosis for women with breast cancer due to delays in detection and treatment. Patient delay is mainly defined as a time gap greater than three months between symptom detection and first medical consultation. Various reasons for this are distrust, disbelief, disregard, fear of breast cancer, higher education level, being employed, absence of support from friends and family, unavailability of specialists, and the socioeconomic and cultural background of patients. Furthermore, symptomatology experience, ethnic origin, and beliefs or perceptions that affect the attitude of patients represent important causal factors of patient delay.

Non-attribution of symptoms to cancer, fear of the disease and treatment, and low educational level were the most frequent causes of patient delay.

System delay is caused by access barriers, such as the long commute to treating healthcare centers or the non-availability of specialized centers. Intrinsic problems of an established healthcare system, like disease management, problems in obtaining or scheduling diagnostic tests, and communication problems between patients and physicians can also cause system delay. Less comprehensive health insurance coverage, older/younger age, and false-negative diagnostic test results were the three most common causal factors of system delay.

Waiting between 31 and 90 days to first treatment after diagnosis with breast cancer may not be a treatment delay and will be acceptable for the patient. Cancer treatment should start very soon after diagnosis, but the above duration gives the person with cancer time to get mentally prepared, decide about the place of treatment, and talk about all their treatment options with the cancer care team, family, and friends. They can then decide what is best for them.

~·⤜⤛·~

Name: Pushpa Tripathi
Age: 38 years
Location: Lucknow

Pushpa Tripathi scraped through her memories to spin out her story, which she claims to be the worst chapter of her life. She said she wanted to caution all the readers, men or women, to never neglect the signs. It is true that cancer doesn't grow in a minute. It pricks you every now and then with its symptoms. But if you choose to ignore your symptoms, little things can take major turns. This is the story of Pushpa Tripathi. I didn't speak about the lump in my breast to my gynecologist when I consulted her about my irregular periods. I waited till it was more pronounced and prominent before I disclosed it to my doctor. Around May 5, 2018, I got a mammogram done. The mammogram did not give a conclusive report, and so the doctor again prescribed an FNAC. The latter cleared the shroud of doubt, and the doctor asked us to immediately consult a specialist either at the Medical College Hospital or PGI, Lucknow. Considering the overwhelming crowd seen in medical colleges, we first chose to go to PGI. We consulted a doctor, who listed out some more diagnostic tests for me.

I underwent a series of tests, such as an X-ray, blood profiling, HIV test, mammogram, FNAC, and biopsy. My biopsy report proved the tumor was cancerous. The doctor had told me that if it was cancer, I would have to undergo surgery, chemotherapy, and radiation therapy accordingly. Cancer was a hefty term to digest. We just could not sit at home without going for a second opinion. Though we were not in the mode of doctor hopping, we wished to confirm the course of treatment. So, we consulted another doctor who referred us to KGMU. Here too, I was advised the same plan of treatment, and I underwent a pre-anesthesia check-up (PAC) for surgery.

While I jot down the chain of events, I wonder if the case would have been the same if I had been vigilant enough. I ignored all the signs time and again just because nothing was hindering my daily life. I had played multiple roles to fit into the prescribed norms. I had been an ideal daughter, a loving and caring daughter-in-law, a conscious mother, and a responsible wife. I was well-informed about every individual in the family: their likes and dislikes, their health issues, their favorite food, and whatnot. While I was drawn into the operation theatre, I looked at all those saddened faces of my family. Their worried mien reflected upon my reluctance toward myself. I had always tried to prove my worth by working harder and harder. I devoted my time to nourishing my family, unbeknownst to the wails of my own body.

I would like to ask all the mothers out there: Do you teach your daughters to check on their bodies regularly? Do you teach them to be unashamed of their bodies?

Leave aside informing about periods. The menstrual cycle is just one part of a woman's life. Do you let your daughter reveal their pain, physical or emotional? No. Time has changed, of course.

A woman is no longer restricted within the courtyard of her home. She works to earn bread for her family, but still, it is she who has to manage the household too. Women are now trading with an undying urge to prove their worth in the outer world as well as in their domestic duties. And while striving for a balance, women forget about the importance of their ailing health. I could have easily gone to the doctor as soon as I found the lump. But I did not. Why? Because I was not taught to check for such symptoms.

I was habituated to adjusting to pain. I was more concerned about every other thing than myself. But then, should I carry this blame all alone? I do not think so. My husband and my whole family loved me; however, my reluctance to confess my problems had blinded them. None in the family was aware of breast cancer symptoms. No one could ever imagine me to be unwell ever. On July 27, 2017, the lump was operated on. I still remember the milieu of relatives who came to show their support.

At around 9.00 in the night, I felt a little hungry and had some tea and biscuits. Around 3.00 a.m., I was fully conscious. The next morning, incidentally, I could do all the morning rituals on my own. It was painful indeed, but I preferred to keep myself going. Within four days, I was allowed to go home. Many of my friends and family paid a visit, and their concern deepened my doubt further. How did I contract the disease? I did not entertain any bad habits, then why me? The surgical incision had some issues and I had delayed suture removal, which delayed my chemotherapy sessions. The doctor prescribed me a series of tests before deciding on my chemo doses. Once ECHO, LFT, and blood profiling were ready, my chemotherapy sessions started. I have been prescribed six cycles of chemotherapy. Looking at the side effects, one can easily comprehend why it is called a battle against cancer. My stomach was queasy all the time. Taste buds were dead; I could not eat anything. Fatigue was my constant companion, along with joint pain.

With every session of chemo, these side effects cropped up and remained for ten days. And by the time I could feel better, another cycle would start. The process started on September 11 and was repeated every 23 days. I remembered the dates as with each cycle, and I realized the importance of health. I understood the significance of being well-informed.

Be well-informed about your body.
Do not hesitate to speak up when you feel something is wrong.

Pushpa tells us that she knew about the lump in her breast but chose not to reveal it to her gynecologist, whom she actually consulted for a different problem regarding her periods. The reason for not disclosing the lump could be many. Innate shyness, fear of the diagnosis, not considering the lump to be a serious issue, or a lack of awareness are just a few of the likely reasons. Pushpa, however, attributes her reticence to a lack of knowledge. And of course, conditioning!

84

She says women and girl children are conditioned from childhood to not speak up about their health issues. As a woman, she is expected to bear any pain and discomfort. After her experience, Pushpa tells women and mothers to encourage and teach their daughters about their bodies. Teach them to identify when something is wrong with their health and seek early medical help. Having gone through the long-drawn cancer treatment with all the anxiety and fear it brings, she is now clear that awareness and education are paramount to a woman's health. And I agree with her. Women need to be taught how to identify a breast lump.

Women need to be encouraged to go for timely screening and clinical breast examination. Early diagnosis and treatment are the keys to becoming cancer-free.

Avail information only from reputed sources. Social media has a lot of misinformation about cancer. Alternative medicine has not been scientifically proven to cure cancer, but instead, the time wasted on these treatments may result in the advancing of the cancer stage, thereby reducing the chances of survival and remission.

Yes, cancer therapy can be long-drawn, but make sure you do not stop your treatment midway. Now, how can you make sure that you pick up signs of breast cancer at an early stage? In the next chapter, let us talk about a very important aspect: breast self-examination.

5

BREAST SELF-EXAMINATION

Be aware of the changes

When you start to feel sick or experience something amiss in your body, the very first person to notice is you. But as we saw in a previous chapter, women often ignore the warning signs in their bodies due to reasons ranging from ignorance to financial constraints. They are immersed in their role as caretakers and do not see themselves receiving care. But breast cancer is one disease where it is imperative that the slightest sign or symptom should not be ignored. We have already seen how the early diagnosis of breast cancer has the multiple benefits of decreased morbidity and mortality and lower cost of treatment. Ignoring your symptoms can turn very costly for the family in the long run. An ounce of prevention is definitely better than a pound of cure, in this case.

This is something that all women need to be educated about. An easy and inexpensive way to monitor for symptoms of breast cancer is the Breast Self-Examination (BSE) technique.

All adolescent girls and women should know BSE. It should be classified as a must-have skill. BSE has the following advantages:

1. It allows a woman to have control over her own health.
2. It provides knowledge to a woman about how her own breast tissue feels.
3. It is a non-invasive and simple procedure.
4. It can detect breast cancer at an earlier stage.

How Can One Learn BSE?

BSE should be included in all health awareness programs for young girls and women. In schools and educational institutions, community health workers, nurses, or doctors can conduct sessions and teach young girls the correct way to do a BSE. Corporates and workplaces can organize yearly programs to raise awareness among their female employees.

Many companies organize these programs to coincide with the Women's Day celebrations or World Cancer Day, or they are held in the month of October every year. Charts with clear pictorial depictions of BSE may be displayed in women's rest areas in workplaces. These can serve as reminders to the women who glance at them.

All health sub-centers, primary health centers, and higher hospitals should have health workers who can teach the correct procedure to the women availing their services. Women who have access to a smartphone can just type in 'Self Breast Examination' in Google.

There are a number of websites that have details of BSE with pictures, and there are a lot of videos on YouTube as well. There are also videos of some of my talks available, or you can access the website of the Lucknow Breast Cancer Support Group.[21]

---

[21] www.lbcsg.com

What Are Some of the Barriers to BSE?

The main deterrent to promoting BSE is the lack of awareness about it. Women should be taught how important this one skill is and how it can help pick up breast problems at a very early stage. They need to be made aware of the numerous benefits of an early diagnosis of breast cancer and the improved survival rates that go with it.

Speaking about breasts is considered taboo in society, making it difficult to involve women in a conversation. Girls are also taught from a young age that it is not right to touch their bodies, and so they are hesitant to learn the technique. There is an inherent embarrassment associated with examining their own breasts. In many homes, the women may not have enough privacy to actually perform a thorough BSE. At times, women do not take the matter seriously and think that BSE is not necessary as they are fine and do not have breast cancer. Another important barrier to practicing BSE is the fear of detecting a lump. The very same symptom they are supposed to identify can scare the women into not performing the examination.

A 2019 study from India looked at the different barriers and facilitators of BSE among rural women[22]. The major barriers to BSE were the false belief that they would not get breast cancer, inadequate knowledge about BSE, and not having enough privacy to perform BSE in their homes. The main sources of information about BSE were television, radio propaganda, and health professionals and social workers in the study. Some responders knew about BSE because a family member, friend, or relative had been diagnosed with breast cancer earlier. It was found that none of the women had accurate knowledge about BSE in the pre-test analysis. Pre-test analysis also showed poor skills in all the responders. We have also conducted a study to identify the present practice of BSE in urban and rural Indian women, including medical and paramedical women.

_____

[22]https://kont.zsf.jcu.cz/pdfs/knt/2019/01/07.pdf

We found that there was relatively more knowledge in the medical group; however, the necessary skills for BSE were suboptimal and did not differ significantly among the women.[23]

The results of this study show that there is a need for adequate knowledge and skills with regard to BSE among rural women. With the help of trained healthcare professionals and nurses, all rural women can use the BSE technique skillfully.

Symptoms of Breast Cancer

The common symptoms of breast cancer are as follows:
1. A mass or lump in the breast or a lump in the armpit.
2. Swelling of all or part of the breast, even if no specific lump is felt.
3. Skin irritation or dimpling.
4. Retraction of the nipple (turned inward).
5. The skin over the nipple or the breast appears red, scaly, or thickened.
6. Nipple discharge, especially on one side, copious or bloodstained.

Role of BSE

Self-examination of the breasts is an important method for detecting the presence of a breast lump or any breast irregularity. It helps to detect the changes suggestive of breast cancer at an earlier stage when there is an increased chance of successful treatment. There is enough evidence to prove beyond doubt that **the earlier the stage of diagnosis in breast cancer, the higher the chance of survival of the patient**. Breast tumors in the early stages have a 97 percent to 100 percent chance of cure.

---

[23]A Survey on Breast Cancer Awareness Among Medical, Paramedical, and General Population in North India Using Self-Designed Questionnaire: a Prospective Study. Indian J Surg Oncol. 2018 Sep;9(3):323-327.

However, this decreases when the tumor spreads (metastasizes) to the lymph nodes in the axilla or to other parts of the body. It would be right to say that BSE helps a woman to detect a breast lump at an earlier stage than she would have if she did not practice BSE. The earliest method to detect breast cancer would be through clinical breast examination and mammography or ultrasonography. BSE and general breast self-awareness keep a woman attuned to the physical appearance and feel of her breasts. They make it easier for her to detect any changes in the external appearance of the breast, such as an increase in the size, skin changes, and retraction of the nipple. Awareness and examination also help in detecting physical changes in the breast that may not be detected externally but can be felt on palpation, such as a lump or swelling that was not previously present, increased nodularity in the breast tissue, and pain on palpation. However, I want to stress that BSE alone cannot play the role in screening for breast cancer. It is important that the other established screening methods, such as regular clinical examination of breasts by trained healthcare professionals and mammography, be implemented as recommended.

When a person is diagnosed to have breast cancer, the cancer is staged depending on the size of the tumor, whether it has spread to the axillary lymph nodes, and whether it has spread to the other parts of the body. Breast cancer is said to spread mainly through the bloodstream to the lungs, long bones, liver, and brain. Stage 1 breast cancer involves a tumor less than 2 cm in size. In stage 2, the tumor size is between 2 cm and 5 cm. It may be difficult for women to identify a tumor less than 5 cm in size, especially in a large breast.

In the King George Medical University Hospital, Lucknow, where I work, and in most Government hospitals or public hospitals, our data depicts that 60 percent of the women with breast cancer presented at an advanced or metastatic stage. This figure is lower in private and corporate hospitals, where only around 20 percent to 25 percent of women present with advanced-stage cancer.

This difference may be due to various factors, such as demographics of the patient population, social status of the patient population, location of the hospital, and catchment area that the hospital caters to. Cost and distance definitely play a significant role in deciding at which stage women present themselves in the hospital. At KGMU, patients have to pay only Rupees 1/- for registration and they can avail of specialist consultation. We not only provide services to the entire state of Uttar Pradesh but also to patients from the neighboring states of Bihar, Uttarakhand, and Madhya Pradesh; patients come to our hospital from Nepal too. Most of our patients hail from rural and semi-urban backgrounds and belong to low- or middle-income status.

I believe that if these women are trained in the right way to perform BSE, they will be able to detect any abnormality externally in their breasts or perceive if there is any difference in how the breast feels. Women may not be able to appreciate small lumps or those located deep in the breast tissue. But they will most likely be able to appreciate the difference in the feel of the breast tissue from the last menstrual cycle. Therefore, although BSE cannot be termed a screening tool for breast cancer, I believe that it has a significant role to play in detecting breast lumps at an earlier stage than they would be otherwise, and help in the earlier presentation of these tumors at the government hospitals.

BSE Procedure

Self-examination of the breast helps a woman become **aware of the shape, size, and feel (consistency) of her breasts and the changes happening over a menstrual cycle**. BSE involves a step-by-step method for a woman to examine her breasts by herself. By looking at and feeling her breasts regularly at 1-month intervals, a woman would be able to identify any change or abnormality in her breasts.

Some important points about BSE:

1. The ideal time for BSE is three to five days after the start of the menstrual cycle. This is because the breasts are physiologically in their most normal phase at this time.
2. It is preferable that BSE is performed monthly, on the same day following the menstrual cycle. For example, if you choose to perform BSE on the third day following the menstrual cycle, it should preferably be performed on the third day every month.
3. BSE is advised in all women above the age of 20 years.

Let us look at the steps involved in BSE. There are two steps: The first step is visual examination and the second step is manual palpation (feeling).

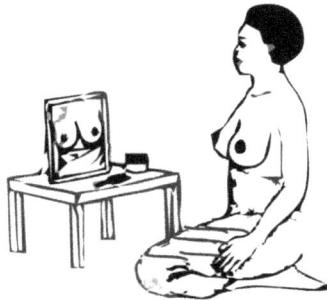

Visualization in front of mirror

Visual Inspection: Stand in front of a large mirror after removing your clothes and undergarments. Ensure that you have a clear view of the entire chest region. This may be done prior to a bath if you have a suitable mirror in the washroom.

First, keep your arms by your side and look for any change in breast size or shape from before. Examine the nipples and the skin over the breast to detect any changes such as reddening, dimpling, etc. Look for retraction of the nipple. Next, compare the size of the breasts on both sides and the position of the nipples. Are they at the same level on both sides? Examine the lower half of the breasts as well. Now, raise both your arms high and look for the same things in both breasts. The third exercise would be to place your hands on your hips and press firmly to flex the muscles of the chest. Again, look for the same changes in both breasts.

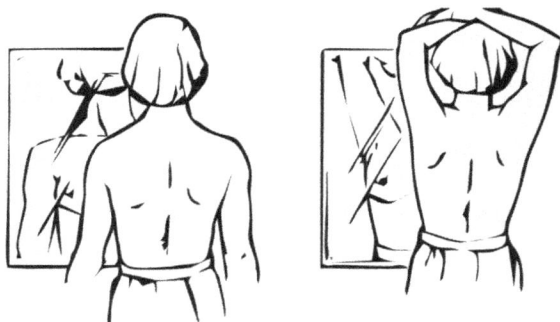

Visualization in front of mirror

Manual Inspection: This involves physically feeling your breasts. Manual inspection is done in two positions: Standing up and lying down. You use your right hand to examine the left breast and vice versa. First, in the standing position, use the pads of the three middle fingers to feel every part of the opposite side breast. Do not use the tips of the fingers. Press gently at first, then use medium pressure, and finally apply firm pressure. Feel for any lumps or swellings, thickened areas, or any other changes. You can move in a circular pattern as you manually feel the breast to avoid missing any area.

Feeling

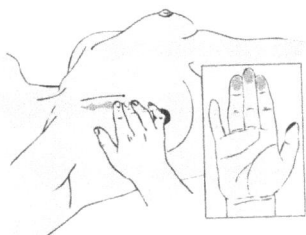

Use the pads of your middle three fingers to feel the texture of your breast.

Your finger pads are the top third of each finger, not the tips.

Self palpation of breast in patterns so that whole breast is palpated

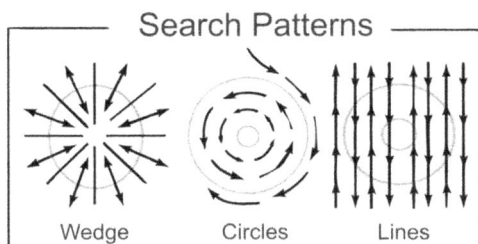

Search Patterns

Wedge   Circles   Lines

Check the areola, the underside of the breast, and the nipples. Feel the tissues under the arm as well by applying pressure. Press the nipples gently to look for any discharge. Repeat the same procedure for the other breast as well. Follow this by performing the examination while lying down. Lying down helps to spread the breast tissues evenly.

This is especially helpful for examining large breasts. To examine the right breast, lie down and place a pillow below your right shoulder.

Raise your right hand and place it behind your head. Now use your left hand to examine and feel the breast just like you did while standing up. Be careful to follow all the steps. Feel the entire breast, the axilla, areola, and nipple. Now exchange the pillow to the other side and proceed to examine your left breast using your right hand.

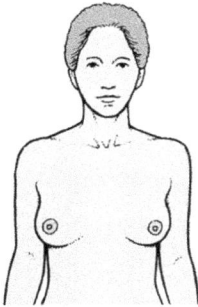

How to Do a Breast Self-Examination

Step 1: While standing in front of the mirror, look at the breast. The breasts normally differ slightly in size. Look for any change in the difference between the breasts and change in the nipple, such as turning inward (an inverted nipple) or a discharge. Look for puckering or dimpling.

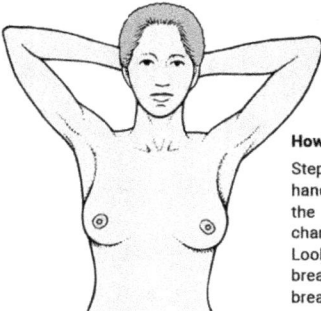

How to Do a Breast Self-Examination

Step 2: Watching closely in the mirror, clasp the hands behind the head and press them against the head. This position helps make subtle changes caused by cancer more noticeable. Look for changes in the shape and contour of the breasts, especially in the lower part of the breasts.

3

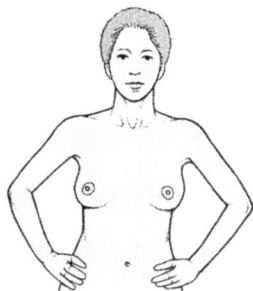

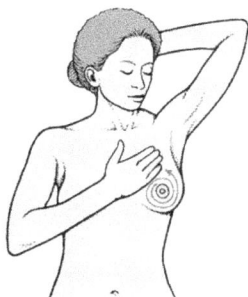

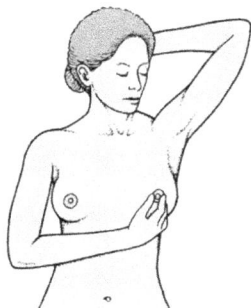

How to Do a Breast Self-Examination

Step 3: Place the hands firmly on the hips and bend slightly toward the mirror, pressing the shoulders and elbows forward. Again, look for changes in shape and contour.

4

How to Do a Breast Self-Examination

Step 4: Raise the left arm. Using three or four fingers of the right hand, probe the left breast thoroughly with the flat part of the fingers. Moving the fingers in small circles around the breast, begin at the nipple, and gradually move outward. Press gently but firmly, feeling for any unusual lump or mass under the skin. Be sure to check the whole breast. Also, carefully probe the armpit and the area between the breast and armpit for lumps.

5

How to Do a Breast Self-Examination

Step 5: Squeeze the left nipple gently and look for a discharge. (See a doctor if a discharge appears at any time of the month, regardless of whether it happens during breast self-examination.)

6

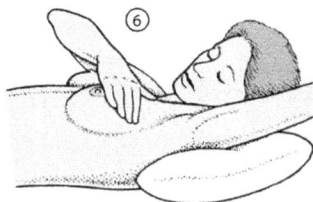

How to Do a Breast Self-Examination
Step 6: Lie flat on the back with a pillow or a folded towel under the left shoulder and with the left arm overhead. This position flattens the breast and makes it easier to examine. Examine the breast as in steps 4 and 5. Repeat for the right breast.

I have listed some of the findings that can be considered significant and that need to be further evaluated by the healthcare practitioner. Do not panic when you feel something different. All breast lumps are not cancer.

1. Any change in the look, feel, or size of the breast.
2. Any change in the nipple.
3. Dimpling or puckering of skin (looks like the skin of an orange).
4. Any lump, swelling, or thickened area.
5. Any discharge from the nipple.
6. Nipple pulled toward any direction.
7. Persistent pain in one spot that does not go away.
8. A rash or skin changes on the nipple.
9. Skin changes, such as redness, dark spots, or increased warmth.

If you find any of the abovementioned signs or symptoms, it is advisable to make an appointment with your surgeon, doctor, or family doctor for further evaluation.

How do you know if you are at risk of developing breast cancer? There are modifiable and non-modifiable risk factors. Five percent of breast cancers are genetic. Males can also develop it. Family history plays a role in increasing the risk of breast cancer. We will see more in detail about that in another chapter.

But I want to stress that all women who are diagnosed with breast cancer do not have a positive family history. A first-degree relative suffering from breast cancer (for example, mother, sister, or daughter) increases your chances of developing breast cancer by almost 50 percent. And if there are two first-degree relatives with the diagnosis, then your chances increase to three times. There are a few other risk factors, such as obesity, which increase one's chances of developing breast cancer. Other risk factors are age above 40, not having any children, history of breast cancer in the other breast, having the first baby above the age of 31, certain gene mutations, and radiation exposure to the chest wall.

Early menarche or late menopause, long-term use of estrogen therapy, cancer in the uterus, ovary, or colon, hormone replacement therapy with estrogen and progesterone, lack of physical activity, and alcohol abuse are also some of the factors that can increase the risk.

At this juncture, I also want to address some of the common myths and false beliefs I have seen among women who come to my clinic. One of the commonly asked queries is, "Can an injury or squeezing or hitting the breasts lead to cancer?" That is not true. Injury to the breast tissue can cause bruising and swelling of the breast, which can be quite painful. But squeezing or pinching the breast or nipple does not cause cancer. Sometimes an injury can lead to a lump in the breast known as fat necrosis; this is a benign condition and not cancer. It is the equivalent of scar tissue forming to heal the injured breast tissues.

Many women attribute their breast cancer to the fine needle aspiration cytology (FNAC) procedure. This is again a false belief. FNAC is a very useful tool for the evaluation of a lump. For further confirmation, core biopsy is needed.

SURVIVOR NOTES

Bidrawati's story highlights how a young woman with a small child from a rural area fought cancer and conquered it. Her story also reminds us of breast cancer awareness and knowledge of BSE.

Name: Bidrawati
Age: 27
Place: Lucknow

I am Bidrawati Yadav and I am 27 years old. I hail from a small village in Uttar Pradesh. These days, I live in Lucknow with my husband Naresh Yadav and my son Tushar, who is 1½ years old. My husband has a retail business, and I have a front desk job in a corporate office. My widowed mother-in-law, too, stays with us and is a great help in looking after my baby and running the home.

I take pride in keeping fit and healthy as everyone knows the front desk staff represents the face of the office to visitors. Here I am with my story of how I faced a sudden turn in my life. The date is clearly etched in my memory—August 2, 2018. It was while in the shower that I accidentally felt a lump in my left breast. My hand stilled, and I could literally feel my heart turning over in my chest. I was a little anxious, and my heart started beating fast. I leaned against the bathroom wall and took a few deep breaths to calm myself. I ran my hand over where I had felt the lump to make sure I did not imagine anything. No, I could definitely feel a small hard lump.

My mind raced back to a health session that had been organized in my office in connection with Women's Day celebrations. A doctor had taken a session on women's health issues, and one of the things they had taught was breast self-examination. At that time, this had made a deep impression on me, and I think this was the reason why I subconsciously examined my breast now and then.

I tried to recall what the doctor had said about breast lumps. The only thing I could recall clearly was the statement, "No Lump Should Be Neglected. Get It Checked Immediately." I immediately shared this with my husband. He was extremely worried hearing my concern, too, but I stood strong and gave him courage. I quoted what I remembered the doctor telling us that day: Breast Cancer is Curable in the Early Stages.

Both of us decided we would not keep this a secret but instead take the counsel of friends. It was amazing to learn that so many people have gone through something similar or have known someone who has. We got a lot of suggestions about where we should go for treatment, but most of them recommended King George's Medical University in Lucknow. We visited the university hospital on August 6, 2018. We were directed to the Department of Endocrine Surgery and met Dr. Anand Mishra for the first time. I think he recognized the worry in our eyes and gave a reassuring smile. He examined me and then asked me to undergo a mammography test. It is like an X-ray of the breast.

After seeing the mammography report, the doctor told us that I would need to undergo a biopsy. A biopsy is a procedure where a small amount of tissue is taken from the lump and sent for pathology testing. A biopsy helps determine whether the breast lump is benign or malignant, whether it is harmless or cancer! The biopsy report came as positive for cancer. The doctor confirmed that I had Stage 2 cancer. Once we had the definitive diagnosis, we started facing a whole new set of confusing questions. What will happen to me? What is the best option now? How to proceed forward? The prospect appeared frightening to my husband and me, and to the others in my family.

However, the doctor's encouraging words helped me a lot at this time. He confidently assured me that I would be able to beat this. Stage 2 cancer is not the end, he said. You need to be brave and positive and have faith in your doctors. His encouraging words brought a ray of hope. I decided I would stand and fight and not get demoralized.

I had to undergo a few more tests and scans to confirm that the cancer was indeed localized and then prepare for surgery. On completion of all the investigations, the doctor went through all my reports. He prescribed some medicines for me and started to plan the surgery. I underwent surgery on September 8, 2018. Following surgery, the doctor told me that I would have to undergo chemotherapy as well. I knew chemotherapy could be an ordeal with all its side effects, but I was prepared mentally to face the challenge. Undergoing chemotherapy is literally like being in a fight. It extracts a lot from the patient, both physically and mentally. My chemotherapy treatment began on December 4, 2018, and went on for nearly six months. My last chemo session was scheduled for May 7, 2019. Dr. Anand personally supervised each of my chemotherapy sessions. His presence gave me a lot of confidence.

Following chemotherapy, I was now asked to undergo radiation therapy (RT). The doctor explained that RT was necessary to ensure that every cancer cell had been removed.

Radiation therapy started on June 27, 2019. Compared to chemo, RT is easier to undergo. I did not have any major side effects except for some skin changes toward the end of my RT sessions. I completed radiation therapy on June 18, 2019. I had 16 cycles of RT.

It was time to meet my doctor again. He carefully perused all my reports and gave me the happy news that I had beaten cancer and was completely rid of it. His words sounded wonderful to my ears. He cautioned me about the importance of regular follow-up in the initial few years to ensure that there is no cancer recurrence.

A periodic check-up is a small price to pay for peace of mind throughout the year! I agreed to be diligent with my follow-up appointments. I am very grateful to all the doctors who were involved with me. I thank them from the bottom of my heart, as without their encouragement, support, and skill, I would not be standing where I am today. The junior doctors, nurses, and other staff from these departments played a major role in helping and encouraging me in every step of my journey.

I want to share what I realized through this incident in my life. Awareness of breast cancer is very important for women. Through the sessions organized by my office, I am thankful that I was made aware of breast cancer and breast self-examination. If I hadn't known these things, I probably would have ignored my lump as nothing significant in the initial stages. When the people in my native village heard the cancer diagnosis, they thought this was the end for me. Some even advised me to make peace with the world and prepare for the worst. This reaction was due to ignorance. They only knew cancer was a dangerous disease. They had no idea about the stages of the disease, advancements in treatment, etc. When they heard that I was cured of cancer after treatment, they were shocked; this was the first time they realized 'Cancer Is Curable.' That is why I tell everyone I meet not to neglect any swelling or lump that they find in the breast or throat. Women need to know that 'Breast Cancer Is Curable In the early Stage!' They should be taught the procedure for breast self-examination.

Women living in rural areas may not go for a mammogram every two or three years as recommended. But they can do a breast self-examination every two weeks. I tell all my friends and acquaintances, "If you find a lump in your breast or throat, please get it tested immediately. You can go to King George's Medical University, Lucknow. The charges are very low, and treatment for the underprivileged is provided free of cost."

Breast self-examination is a life-saving skill.

Bidrawati had some awareness about breast cancer and the importance of self-examination. This led to her cancer being diagnosed early. Early diagnosis of breast cancer has many advantages for the patient. Not only is the survival rate better, but the treatment is also easier. The cure rate is almost 100 percent. And for poor or underprivileged patients, much of the treatment will get covered under the various schemes of the Government.

With advanced-stage breast cancer, not only is the morbidity higher, the cost of treatment goes up as well. To start with, patients have to travel to tertiary cancer care centers for treatment and the associated expenses increase accordingly. In addition, many of the therapies for advanced-stage cancer are not covered under any of the schemes and hence these are not free. Patients have to look for funding for targeted therapies and innovative treatment modes.

Name: Rita Chaturvedi
Age: Undisclosed
Place: Lucknow

Cancer does not appear suddenly; it slowly takes root in the body. I am Rita Chaturvedi, a cancer survivor. I am working as Assistant Chief Technical Officer & Nodal Officer of Information Technology and Infrastructure in the National Bureau of Fish Genetic Resources. At first, I wondered, "How could this be?"

There was nothing to suggest that this would be my fate.

I quickly learned that the question of "why me" is unanswerable. It makes no difference. It was now my responsibility to live as long and normally as possible, or so I believed. Cancer gradually robs you of your life. It starts by stealing your health. Then you lose your time and career, and finally, your future is taken away. It can even take your friends or family members, which is horrifying. Those who cannot cope with the diagnosis of metastatic breast cancer fade away, out of your life. After all, how long can you expect people to stick around when your diagnosis makes them uncomfortable? Under these new conditions, you will build some new relationships magically. Kindness can be found in places you did not expect and from those you did not know. You are drawn into the circle of camaraderie and comfort.

People will send you greeting cards, provide food, and offer hugs. There will be those who will volunteer to help you with housework, transport you to appointments, and even laugh at your silly jokes. You will find that some value you more than you ever knew, and you will realize that they are the only ones who matter. These are the ones who encourage you and boost up your spirits, and your dread of the disease fades as the years roll by. It has not always been easy for me since I was diagnosed, but you will notice that I mentioned nobody gave up on me, not even my doctor, who was the most important person in my life. There was no set end date for my treatment, and I was expected to make progress at all times.

In 2016, I went to meet my doctor for a check-up. At that time, he asked me to get a mammogram done, and seeing the report, he prescribed some medications. After two years, my symptoms appeared again in February 2018. I went back to my doctor, and this time after the physical check-up, he did not prescribe any medicines but referred me for a pathology test instead. My husband accompanied me as I went for the mammography and the FNAC tests. The FNAC report was not very encouraging, and I was beginning to feel uneasy and anxious.

My doctor informed me that I would probably require surgical treatment.

However, as he was not a surgeon, he referred me for treatment to another doctor. I was warned that the cost might be up to 4 to 5 lakh rupees. We then forwarded my reports to another doctor who was at that time the Joint Director of Uttar Pradesh's Samaj Kalyan Vibhag. He advised us to go straight from the office to the outpatient department (OPD) at King George's Medical University (KGMU), and not anywhere else. He said it is better to get there early than take the risk of my case being mismanaged in a private hospital. In which case, I would end up going to KGMU in an advanced stage with a decreased chance of recovery. Some of my colleagues even suggested that I travel to Delhi for further treatment. Well, my husband took me to KGMU for further assessment, and this was when we met the consultant in the OPD on March 19, 2018.

After the physical check-up, the doctor at KGMU asked us to get a biopsy gun from the medical store. He assured us that after performing the biopsy, he would be able to provide us with some clarity and clear all our doubts.

I underwent a core biopsy of the lump. I was also asked to undergo some blood tests and repeat the mammography along with ultrasonography of the breast and a 2D echocardiography. These tests were for confirmation of my diagnosis and also to check my fitness for surgery.

I also underwent a PET CT. It was a scary procedure. Finally, with all the reports, we went to meet the doctor again at the OPD of KGMU. I was hoping and praying that my reports would be normal. However, it was Cancer! I was advised to get a chemo port inserted. This would make it easy to inject my chemotherapy medicines and it would not be necessary to look for a vein each time.

At this time, our home situation was a bit chaotic as well. My father-in-law was not keeping well, and he was also bed-ridden. My daughter was in Class X and her ICSE Board Examinations were fast approaching. My husband and I were already quite disturbed, and now my condition worsened the situation further.

Both of us were left feeling quite helpless about how to care for everyone in the family. Finally, we decided that it was best to let people know about the situation. So once my treatment regimen was definite, we informed our friends and relatives. We were sure that they would all be concerned and lend a helping hand when necessary. We went back to see the doctor in the KGMU OPD in May 2018, after making all of our decisions. My first chemotherapy session was on May 18, 2018, at 9.00 a.m. I remember there were three patients on that day, all women, and the doctor and his staff carried out the chemo port placement while talking to us in such a way that we did not even notice the procedure. Then, on May 19, 2018, I was admitted to the hospital and had my first chemo treatment. The medical staff administered the chemo medications to me via the chemo port. The session went smoothly and I was told to return in 21 days for the next cycle of chemotherapy.

In the event of any difficulty, we were welcome to contact the senior resident through WhatsApp, and he promised to help in any way he could. The smiling faces of all the physicians and staff members here, while they talked and interacted with the patients, helped to boost our confidence at the time. During my various chemotherapy sessions, I have witnessed the doctors personally help obtain chemo drugs for underprivileged people. The physicians here are really dedicated. We only work at a 9–5 job; however, the doctors here work from 9.00 a.m. to 10.00 p.m. I am sure they had night duties as well. The patients admitted here for chemotherapy are provided with a healthy breakfast, lunch, and dinner. My last chemo took place on September 1, 2018.

Realizing suddenly that your time on earth is probably going to be less than what you had anticipated makes you see things in a whole new light. It became important to me that I should make an effort to assist others who may be in the same situation as I was. Before my diagnosis, I had no idea of metastatic breast cancer or its deadly prognosis. I set out to create a social media presence so that I could share and educate others about my experiences.

I started writing and sharing about my diagnosis on social media and interacting with other women who had breast cancer in various ways. After the chemo sessions, I was advised to undergo surgery. I was immediately reduced to tears on hearing this. Sir reassured me and gave me hope by boosting my confidence. He said that when I had already crossed the difficult days of multiple chemotherapy cycles, why should I be afraid of surgery!

In the meantime, the date for my surgery was fixed for October 1, 2018. I was admitted a day before to complete the pre-surgery check-up and tests. My sister, brother, and sister-in-law had come to stay at our home, and their presence helped relieve our anxiety about looking after the home. Following my surgery, I was discharged from the hospital on October 4, 2018, and we went home. At this time, we suffered a loss in the family; my father-in-law breathed his last on October 25, 2018. We next had to submit the surgery report and the pathology report to the Professor at the radiotherapy department.

After checking my reports, I was scheduled to undergo 16 sessions of radiotherapy. My radiotherapy treatment took place from 05.12.2018 to 27.12.2018.

By the Almighty's grace, I recovered. I am now cancer-free, which is incredible! My mental strength and the tireless efforts of the doctors and the staff are what allowed me to reclaim my future. I take a cautious stride forward, but I will never forget what cancer taught me. When you have metastatic cancer, you must live in the present. The future is nothing more than a dream, and the past is nothing more than vapors. Not just for you, but for everyone, now is all there is. This is the secret of life.

There is great progress being made in cancer treatment every day. Perjeta, a monoclonal antibody, was not on the market when I was diagnosed. It is an extremely expensive drug but plays a vital role in certain types of metastatic cancers that are positive for a receptor called HER2Neu. It is given in addition to surgery, chemo, and radiation therapy, with very good results.

Now I visit the KGMU OPD for routine follow-up, and I continue to take some medicines daily. It was mentally difficult for me to accept the diagnosis of metastatic cancer at first. Here are six things I wish I had known when I was younger. It is my hope that this information will be useful to those who have just been diagnosed with metastatic breast cancer.

Recognize that not all cases of metastatic breast cancer are the same. My friend's mother died of metastatic breast cancer. She had the sickness for three years, and it was a rough three years for her. I thought that my experience would probably be the same as hers, but her mother had an illness that was aggressive and widespread. As for my disease, I have a small number of bone metastases that have been rather stable over the last five years. Of course, therapies have evolved during the last three decades. People with minimal bone involvement can live a long life with their condition. I am fortunate to be one of the lucky ones. Keep in mind that your results may vary. You would think that a diagnosis of metastatic breast cancer entails major changes, but this is not always the case.

I see my oncologist every two months, but I continue to do everything I did before I was diagnosed with stage 4 breast cancer. Every day, I go to work. I am a traveler. I am willing to help others. My family and I spend time together. That is not true for everyone with metastatic breast cancer, but do not ever give up!

The problem is with the tissue. The key to knowing treatment choices is your pathology report. Your ER/PR and HER2Neu status are your guideposts, although other considerations (age, past therapy, etc.) must be taken into account. If you have had breast cancer before, ask for a fresh biopsy if it is possible. Cancers can evolve and do so! Get the assistance you require. So, if the stress and emotions are getting to you, speak out. Consult your doctor for assistance. Anti-anxiety drugs are useful, and most cancer clinics have counselors on staff or may direct you to one in your area. I am very grateful to my family members who always stood by me through this difficult time and kept encouraging my husband and me.

I am very indebted to my colleagues at my office who not only supported and encouraged me during this difficult time, but also helped us financially. Finally, to all of you, the readers, who are reading my story:

If you had asked me five years ago what I would be doing and how I would live, I would have given you an answer that would be light years away from what I would say now. Sometimes, I do get angry that I have to keep going for follow-up and must continue with medications to keep going. If I claimed that everything now was hearts and sparkles, I would be lying. But I consider myself fortunate that I get to work with my friends daily, and I am confident that I will leave a legacy that my kid will be proud of and pass down to his children, should I pass away before they meet me. I would love to help out with the kids. I would like to be able to accompany my spouse on his travels. With cancer, you realize that these kinds of activities are not guaranteed. There is a valuable lesson to be learned in terms of how you live your daily life. When you are diagnosed with cancer, just remember that your life is not over and that cancer is just one aspect of your life. You can still do whatever you want.

Cancer is not the end; live life to the fullest.

Yes, the fight against cancer is long and hard at times, as you can see from Rita's experience. But the important point is to never give up hope. When you take the right steps toward your treatment, the journey of hope begins. There are many others to lend a hand, be it your doctor and his treating team or your circle of family and friends. Take the help offered, and remember, a bad day does not signify the end. You may have to face many difficult days before you win over the disease. But with hope and perseverance, it can be done. Given the importance of early detection of a breast lump, I would say that our health centers should play a greater role in regularizing and promoting the culture of BSE. Just like there are Apps available that help men and women in their pursuit of health by providing support and timely reminders, one can be developed for breast cancer awareness as well. It can send reminders to women in vulnerable age groups about BSE, clinical breast examination, and mammography. A text message from the healthcare provider or the family doctor can be quite effective as well.

In the work sector, too, organizations can make it mandatory for their women employees to learn the skills of BSE and for those above the age of 40 to undergo mammography every two years. Basically, information regarding BSE must be effectively shared with the public through the media. Sessions to teach the correct way of performing BSE may be arranged in educational institutions and workplaces. To do this in an effective way, the various healthcare workers and medical staff must have adequate in-service training on these subjects first. A concerted effort on all our parts can definitely increase awareness about breast cancer and aid in the early diagnosis of the same. A question that remains in every woman's mind once she has been diagnosed and has started the various treatment regimes for breast cancer would be, "Can I lead a normal life once my treatment is complete?" Let us look at the challenges that a breast cancer survivor has to face in the next chapter.

6

THROUGH A BREAST CANCER SURVIVOR'S EYES

The survivor's perspective

How does it feel when you have got through the cancer treatment? For months, or maybe even a few years, your mind would have been filled with thoughts of death, survival, treatments, and expenses. But finally, the day arrives when your doctor tells you, you have been cured of cancer and your treatment is now complete.

Yes, the relief is beyond belief, but can everything go back to the way it was? A person who completes a course of cancer therapy that included the whole gamut of surgery, chemotherapy, radiation therapy, immunotherapy, and targeted therapy is nothing short of a soldier returning home from a hard-fought war. Along with the exhilaration, there is extreme exhaustion as well.

In his poem titled 'Fear,' the writer Kahlil Gibran describes the thoughts of a river before merging into the sea thus: *"It is said that before entering the sea a river trembles with fear. She looks back at the path she has traveled, from the peaks of the mountains, the long winding road crossing forests and villages."*

Yes, the journey would have been long and arduous and when you look back, you realize what a tough path you have traveled. Will you have the time to rest and recuperate after your ordeal? Unfortunately, most often, women realize that they have to pick up the threads of their life almost immediately. If one is a wife and a mother, the duties of the home and hearth beckon. You feel guilty for not having taken care of the family for these many months, and so plunge yourself back into your role wholeheartedly. The same applies to the return to your professional life as well. After months of availing of sick leave, you now want to get back to your job.

But in reality, how easy is this return to 'normalcy?' Indeed, can everything be as before the treatment? The fact is that your mind and body need time and care in returning to the life you left behind when you were diagnosed with breast cancer. It is important that you give yourself the time and the space to recover. There should be no hurry to get back to 'normal.' Life after cancer therapy can be a daunting prospect, and you have to learn how to deal with the 'new normal.' Who is a cancer survivor? Let us see what the term surviving cancer actually means. Being a cancer survivor can mean different things. The most straightforward meaning would be having no signs of cancer after completing the treatment. A cancer survivor can also be a person who is living with cancer, through the diagnosis, treatment, and after. The terms used to differentiate these different phases are acute survivorship, extended survivorship, and permanent survivorship.

- Acute survivorship stands for the period from the diagnosis of breast cancer till the end of the initial treatment. During this time, the focus is mainly on treating cancer.

- Extended survivorship starts at the end of the initial treatment and goes through for some months thereafter. During this period, the focus is on the effects of cancer and cancer therapy.

- Permanent survivorship is the timeframe years after the cancer treatment. The chances of recurrence are very low. The focus here is on treating the long-term effects of cancer and cancer therapy.

In short, we can say that cancer survivorship starts right from the time of diagnosis. It lasts through the entire life thereafter. Cancer survivorship can mean different things to different people. And consequently, people may find different areas challenging when facing life after the diagnosis of breast cancer. I am providing here a broad perspective of the different challenges a cancer survivor is likely to face and how they can overcome these challenges.

Physical Challenges

Many cancer patients notice that their physical appearance is quite changed at the end of their treatment. Hair loss occurs as a side effect of chemotherapy. The hair regrowth may be very different from what you had before. You are likely to feel tired easily. Many patients experience excessive weight loss that alters their appearance considerably. These changes can give rise to considerable anxiety in the survivors. They may be hesitant to go out and face people because of their changed appearance. Patients also experience disturbances in their sleep patterns after the intense treatments they have undergone. Lack of adequate sleep can lead to tiredness.

The best way to deal with these issues is to start following a healthy diet. Take the help of a nutritionist or a dietician and begin to eat healthily. The changes will not happen in a day. It will be a slow process, but you will slowly regain the lost weight. Also, the nutritionist will help you make appropriate dietary choices that can help restore health to your hair and skin.

When you have received chemotherapy, steroid therapy, or hormonal therapy as part of breast cancer treatment, you are prone to develop a condition called osteoporosis. In this condition, the bones may become thin and weak, and you may experience bone pain. Your doctor will prescribe calcium and Vitamin D supplements to counteract this. You can also opt to eat foods rich in calcium. Another recommendation is to take part in some daily physical activity, such as walking or cycling. It need not be strenuous, but make it a regular habit. Be gentle with yourself. Many of the targeted therapies and radiation therapy to the chest wall region can lead to heart problems.

You might experience irregularity in your heartbeat, damage to the heart muscle, or thickening of the pericardium (outer covering of the heart). Check with your doctor about any of these problems and find out how often you need to go for cardiac evaluations as a follow-up. Chemotherapy and radiation therapy to the chest area can cause lung problems as well. There may be residual inflammation and thickening of the lining of the lungs, causing breathing difficulties. This might require monitoring as well.Lymphedema in the arm is one of the common sequelae of breast cancer surgery, and it can be a very distressing one as well. There is no permanent cure for this, but it can be managed effectively by following your doctor's instructions carefully with regard to exercise, massaging, etc. The use of customized arm sleeves helps in keeping the swelling under control by exerting constant pressure on the arm. Be meticulous in performing the arm exercises that have been recommended by the physiotherapist and use the arm sleeves every day without fail.

Mental Challenges

From the time a woman learns she has breast cancer, she is on an emotional roller coaster. Each day brings more thoughts and fears crowding into her mind. She is waiting for the time when she can complete her treatment and get on with her life.

But to her shock, these mental hurdles continue to occur even after being termed a cancer survivor. What can one do?

The commonest fear in women who have completed their breast cancer treatment successfully is recurrence. This is the question foremost in their minds: Can I get cancer again? This question, if not addressed, can affect the quality of life to a very large extent. So, if you are a breast cancer survivor, it is important that you talk to your oncologist about this possibility. Your treating doctor will inform you about the chances of recurrence and follow-up monitoring.

The doctor or the healthcare worker will tell you about specific signs and symptoms you need to look out for. They will also tell you how often you need to go in for these follow-up assessments and the tests that will be done as part of this process. All these go toward catching a recurrence early should it occur. Therefore, if you are regular with your follow-up, you can set your mind at ease the rest of the time.

Women who have crossed the breast cancer bridge successfully find themselves unable to concentrate or remember things. They find that they have attention and memory issues. There are many terms used for this condition: cancer-related cognitive impairment, chemo brain, chemo fog, to name a few. Whatever it is called, it can be a very distressing condition to have. You suddenly find your dreams of getting back to your regular self dashed. You find that you are not able to concentrate on what you are doing. You still need someone to help you with chores you used to perform effortlessly. You may find it difficult to even complete simple daily activities at home. If you are facing any of these problems post-completion of therapy, bring it to the attention of your healthcare team or doctor. They will help you overcome these issues.

Often, these symptoms can occur alongside a condition called cancer-related fatigue. The woman finds herself facing extreme tiredness and a lack of energy or enthusiam to do any work. Cancer-related fatigue is not the same as the fatigue experienced by a healthy person. Here the person experiences extreme mental, emotional, and physical tiredness.

This fatigue can remain for months or even years after completion of the treatment. It can seriously affect a person's life and their relationships with friends and family. Women suffering from cancer-related fatigue find it extremely difficult to return to their jobs. If you have any of the symptoms of this condition, make sure you inform your doctor. Some women experience intense anxiety and depression after completing treatment for breast cancer. This can be because they are unsure about their future. For so many months or years, their lives revolved around cancer and the treatment.

Now, all of a sudden, they are overwhelmed by the change. Joining a support group for cancer patients and survivors can help greatly. You can talk to other women who have undergone the same problems and learn how they coped. Your doctor might recommend seeing a psychologist who can help you with cancer-oriented therapy sessions. These psychologists are trained to understand the mindset of cancer survivors and can best help them.

A lot of women have rage and anger in them, which is common among cancer survivors. This anger can stem from a feeling of helplessness or from thoughts of "why me"? They may be resentful of the fact that they had to undergo the illness or that they had to undergo a mastectomy. They may be angry because they lost out in their professional field as a result of breast cancer. It is normal to have these kinds of thoughts and feelings. But they should not overshadow everything else. When you find yourself completely preoccupied with these resentful thoughts and you find that you are spending the entire day mourning the time lost to cancer, it is time to get help. Your doctor can suggest psychologists who can help you overcome these thoughts. Yoga and meditation can help you overcome anger as well.

After undergoing the arduous course of treatment, the women may often be subjected to mood swings. The end of therapy and being termed cancer-free is supposed to bring happiness, but it does not. One of the reasons can be survivor's guilt. This term may not be well-recognized in our country.

Basically, the woman feels she does not deserve to be a survivor, she does not deserve to live. Women who suffer from survivor's guilt often blame themselves for getting cancer. It is important for these women to open up and talk about their feelings, either with their healthcare provider or in a support group. If you are having these kinds of thoughts, it is important to acknowledge your feelings and speak out about them. Dealing with your feelings openly will help you heal soon. Emotional numbness is another sequel to the cancer journey. After being through this tumultuous period of diagnosis and treatment, the cancer survivor chooses to emotionally shut down.

They feel unable to handle any more intense emotions. The immense amount of pain that these women underwent is the reason for this lack of ability to feel any more emotions. This is not a good place to be. If you feel emotionless after being declared cancer-free, you definitely need a psychologist's help. They will talk you through your feelings and help you to open up. Keeping yourself from any kind of emotional investment can make you lose your interest in life very soon.

Professional Challenges

Getting back to work after completing cancer therapy is not as easy as it sounds. Some women continue to work through their time of therapy, taking time off only when required. But some job profiles may not be suitable for that sort of adjustment, and you might have had to take time off during the course of your treatment. Going back to work can be a happy event, and it will definitely boost your self-worth and confidence. Going back to work helps reinforce the thought that you can still be a contributing member of the family and society.

If you have missed being around your colleagues and coworkers, getting back can make you feel less lonely and definitely boost your spirits. However, you will face some difficulties in the initial days.

You may find that you get tired easily and cannot immediately cope with full-time work. Or you may find it difficult to concentrate and focus on the job. You have to be patient with yourself in these situations. Talk to your boss or senior about various options that you can take. Can you start with flexi-hours or part-time work? Can you work from home for a few months? At work, you may face different reactions from your colleagues. Most will be understanding and will offer to help you in any way they can. However, there may be some people who are resentful or uncomfortable around you. The diagnosis of cancer can make some people very uncomfortable, and you have to be prepared to face that. Share about your health only if you are comfortable talking about your journey; otherwise, politely decline to talk by informing them that you do not wish to speak about it. It is not a must that you tell your entire story to everyone at the workplace.

Also, speak about it only if invited to do so. Cancer survivors who suffer from a negative body image after their treatment find it doubly difficult to get back in the public eye. They feel that cancer has taken a toll on their physical appearance and they might be judged by people for not looking their best. Women who have undergone a mastectomy, especially, can benefit from prosthetic breast support. Some women find that using a wig after chemotherapy gives them more confidence in going out. It is important that you do whatever it takes to make you feel better and more confident. Wear the wig till your hair grows out. But some women have found this period a chance to experiment with short hairstyles and loved it.

Sexual and Fertility Issues

Following the various therapies and surgery in the treatment of breast cancer, the woman often feels like her femininity has been damaged. The breast is perceived as a symbol of femininity, and the loss of a breast hits a woman hard when she undergoes a mastectomy.

Moreover, once the diagnosis of cancer has been established, there may be a decrease or cessation of physical relationship with her spouse or partner. Initially, this may be due to the loss of interest caused by the rigors of treatment and its side effects. However, many women experience changes in their sexual function or sex drive caused by cancer and cancer treatment. The physical changes in the body can affect their self-image, self-confidence, and sense of attractiveness. Hormonal treatments can give rise to problems such as vaginal dryness. These problems can be resolved if you speak to your doctor openly. You will be referred to the right person or therapist who can help you. Cancer therapy can affect the fertility of a woman. The woman may have many doubts about whether they can conceive after cancer treatment. Specialists in reproductive endocrinology and infertility can help these women.

SURVIVOR NOTES

Name: Suraiya Bano
Age: Undisclosed
Location: Lucknow

Women often are strong enough to just whisper at iron bars and make them bend out of their way, like the craziest magic. A woman's love can fix souls, fix brains, and cure us all. But when it comes to a woman's own health, she keeps everything on the backburner.

My name is Suraiya Bano, and I define myself as a breast cancer survivor. My story is about the struggle of trying to overcome the social stigma associated with breast removal.

Cancer, for me, is a malicious cage where every patient wears the masks of coping and normality. The disease is outrageous and inflicts pain on every aspect of life. There were times when I was emotionally starved and physically exhausted.

My soul crumbled into pieces while plodding through the darkest lane of my life. Every passage carried a jargon I could neither pronounce nor fathom. However, I am not here to scare any of my readers with the umpteen number of rounds I had to make around the hospitals or how much money I had to spend. As women, we all learn to hide our pain and pretend that everything is fine. And as my body was bound by breast cancer, I began to feel cold deep inside me as I longed to escape the pain of isolation and social stigma. I have seen people's empathy withering on seeing the financial burden my treatment would bring. I received innumerable suggestions on breast cancer treatment from every corner of the world, but hilariously, none of those could weave any miraculous effect on my cancer. It was August of 2017. My left breast felt different than usual. It was hardened, and as I pressed, I felt a lump.

The lump was hard and a little painful. Initially, I tried to overlook this, but the discomfort continued. Something was not right within me. I was always tired, and my appetite had gone down drastically. I informed my husband and he took me to KGMU for a consultation. A series of tests were done and the doctor concluded that the lump in my left breast was cancerous. The term *Cancer* parades an incorrigible fear. No sane human can feel normal after hearing that name. I was crestfallen. We live in a society where every good thing is served to the man first, and the woman gets only the leftovers. A man with an illness is taken care of, but when a woman becomes ill, she is considered a burden.

The doctor's words nettled my innards. So, was I going to die immediately, or was I to be bedridden for the rest of my life? Perhaps the doctor could read my predicament. He asked me not to worry as he was there to help me get rid of this vicious disease. None of us has seen God, but today if I am alive and leading a normal life, it is because of the doctors like Dr. Anand Mishra in the endocrine surgery department of KGMU. They are akin to Gods in disguise. I consider myself lucky to have gotten in touch with Dr. Mishra at the right time. Being a woman, the removal of my breast seemed like losing my worth as a human.

What would people say? How would I look at myself in the mirror? My chest will be as flat as a man's. The dark pall of doubt filled my mind, and I could already sense the disgust of others when they knew about my mastectomy. I was slowly drowning in the ocean of self-deprecation.

However, I could not escape the operation. I underwent surgery on October 20, 2017, and my left breast was surgically removed. The next road to cross in my treatment was the chemotherapy sessions. Around November 16, 2017, my chemotherapy started and I had to sit for six sessions. It was further followed by 16 sessions of radiotherapy, and the treatment concluded in 2018. Yes, the treatment lasted for nearly a year. After all, it was not the common cold, but rather breast cancer, the most melancholic of all diseases.

Today, as I lead a normal life like any other woman, I would like to pen down my thoughts and feelings regarding the social stigma associated with breast cancer. We live in a society where a woman is considered an emblem of beauty, a machine for reproduction, and a caretaker of everyone. I am a woman from Lucknow, and my view is probably myopic toward the global scenario of breast cancer survivors. However, with my limited knowledge, I can tell you that in most patients, the diagnosis of breast cancer is made when the disease has reached an advanced stage. But why? The most common reasons would be a lack of awareness and negligence, while the fear of social stigma comes a close second. Misattribution of the cause and ignorance of the nature of the disease play key roles in shaping our mentality. Illiterate women or less educated people perceive a higher level of stigma associated with the disease. Simply put, education brings health awareness. But then, we cannot overlook another crucial perspective of society. A young woman goes through constant social evaluations about her body, and thus such a drastic effect on the breast is distressing. On the contrary, an older woman would have experienced the changes in her body and would be psychologically more equipped to deal with a breast loss or change in appearance.

As I recall my experience, this long course of treatment indeed cured me; however, I developed an anxiety disorder, adjustment problems, and above all, signs of chronic depression. It was not due to the unbearable pain of losing a part of my body or the pain of the radiation doses. It was more about what people would think of me. No hair on my head, wrinkled skin wrapped around my bony frame, pale as a ghost, I moved around like a lifeless creature under the unforgiving gaze of those around me. And honestly, it was not only me who harbored such thoughts. Most of the women who face this battle against cancer tend to think this way. The societal stigma is so strong that we often feel bereft of any love. No matter how much my husband and family supported me, I always remained apprehensive.

Removal of a breast is potentially stigmatizing for a woman. It causes social isolation and sexuality concerns. And in every way possible, we often fall into the pit of self-blame. The constant worry of death keeps interfering with our family responsibilities. We are bestowed with different kinds of reactions. Some are shocked, some get saddened, while some disperse pity. The disgrace associated is so transparent that people are often reluctant to disclose information. There are women who wish to bask under the illusion that all is fine. The breast is more of a symbol of femininity, and thus, the thought of removing it leads to low self-esteem. Losing one's feminine physical charisma is the biggest stigma linked with breast cancer.

But here I am, a middle-aged woman, walking with my head held high. I am not ashamed to talk about my disease. Yes, I was diagnosed with cancer of the breast and I underwent mastectomy (surgical removal of the breast) performed by a group of able doctors. One of the most significant decisions of my life was to go to a knowledgeable doctor who was confident to give me a normal life. The disease indeed brought a physical burden and psychological stress, which were further compounded by religious beliefs and practices. I could never sit alone and was always scared that my family would abandon me.

My diagnosis had emotional ramifications on my family members. I could never discern whether they were concerned about my recovery or worried about losing me. I felt like every eye was watching my deteriorating condition. Still, I had overcome every bit of it. As the years passed by, I realized I was never alone. Every woman, whether she is working or is a homemaker, runs her household thinking she is the safest inside the walls of the house. But believe me, it is not so. We women are not safe anywhere. We are under the constant scrutiny of society. We all thrive under pain— the pain of societal norms and prejudices. Misogyny strangulates us. Patriarchy dictates to us. And cancer is a disease. It comes to kill you. Living for yourself and your loved ones is more significant than having a beautiful body.

I survived a dreadful disease, and here I confess to leading a life basking in the glory of hope. My body is beautiful in whatever way it is. None can question my integrity or femininity because of the absence of a breast. I was a woman, am a woman, and shall remain a woman till my last breath. My womanhood lies in the love I shower and the hope I disperse, and no despicable taint like social stigma can humiliate me in this life. We women cannot be placid like calm waters all the time. We must become rational creatures and live a life beyond social dictates.

Your feminine identity is in who you are, and losing a breast does not diminish it in any way.
Womanhood lies in the love we shower and the hope we disperse.

Suraiya Banu talks candidly about the many challenges that she faced in her fight against cancer. She is very much aware of the social stigma attached to the diagnosis of cancer. Her thoughts from the time of her diagnosis portray clearly what a woman is likely to face in our society. The fear of standing out, the fear of being a drain of the family's resources, and the inability to look after the family while undergoing treatment are some of the very real concerns.

She is aware of the fact that many women do not disclose that they have a problem, a lump in the breast, until the tumor has reached an advanced stage. The reasons are clear to her. A woman who is sick is considered a burden in our society. They are looked upon with pity and sometimes derision. Suraiya is aware that treatment of cancer can have drastic sequelae, such as a change in the physical appearance and loss of hair. Mastectomy is considered a loss of the very symbol of her femininity, and she has to face that. Along with fighting the disease, she was also battling anxiety and depression. But she is aware that her mental problems are not caused so much by the painful surgery and the radiation therapy or the actual fact of losing her breast as by her fears of how she will be perceived by society. After the breast was removed, she realizes that her fears have indeed come true.

Although her husband and her family give their whole support, she still shrinks from the judgmental gaze of society.

However, she ends her story on a note of hope. Despite how society might view her after the surgery and treatment, she is alive and hopeful of the future. She says there is much to look forward to, having fought and won over dreadful breast cancer. She is proud of her scars and proud of the way she fought her way out. Her words to women everywhere can be a beacon of light. Women should not be placid and calm always. Sure, these are the traits that are considered desirable in a woman, but there are times when you have to stand up for yourself and fight your way through.

Women's health always takes a backseat in patrilineal societies the world over. Women rarely have the autonomy to make decisions in these societies. Childcare and household duties are more difficult when you do not have autonomy. All decisions regarding health are made by the men in the family. Women in these societies have lesser access to healthcare resources than women in matrilineal societies.

Name: Azmi Siddique
Age: 34
Location: Lakhimpur

I am Azmi Siddique. I am 34 years old, and I live in a small city called Lakhimpur, in the district of Lakhimpur Kheri. It is the largest district in Uttar Pradesh, India, and shares a border with Nepal. I am married, and I have an 8-year-old daughter. I have been working as a teacher in a local primary school for nine years, and life was pretty much uneventful and smooth for us. I enjoyed my work and loved interacting with my students. My extended family included my parents, parents-in-law, aunts, uncles, and cousins. Most of them lived in Lakhimpur or nearby places. My whole life revolved around my family. But my idyllic life was to receive a jolt in August 2020. I had felt a small swelling in my left breast. Initially, I was not sure and thought it must not be significant.

However, on examining a week later, I felt the swelling again, and this time it seemed a little bigger. I panicked and confided in my best friend, who was also my colleague. She calmed me down and took me to her relative, who was a doctor. The doctor examined me and confirmed that it was indeed a swelling and that I must get it investigated immediately.

That evening after returning from the clinic, I told my husband. He was stunned for a moment but immediately said, "Don't worry. We will go and get all the tests done." He encouraged me and gave me courage. I underwent an FNAC test and ultrasound examination of the breast. The tests confirmed that the swelling was malignant. I was given the diagnosis of breast cancer stage 2. Now came the most difficult days of my life. I was scared and confused about what I should do next. My family would have to be told, but I knew they would be terribly distressed to hear this too.

My husband and I discussed this endlessly, and we decided to disclose the news to our parents and siblings because we needed their moral support at this difficult time. That is the wonderful thing about families. In a crisis, they will rally around and support you with their love and presence.

When my family members heard about my diagnosis, they too were shocked and upset initially. But they soon recovered from the initial shock and stood by to help us. We started discussing the various treatment options. A few friends from my workplace knew about it, and they too gave their suggestions. It made me feel a lot better to know that so many people were there to support me. Of course, we knew the treatment had to start as soon as possible to prevent it from spreading further. I finally decided to get treated at the Medical College Hospital as it was well equipped and had very experienced doctors working there. I took an appointment to meet Dr. Anand Mishra, who worked in the Department of Endocrine Surgery. I will never forget that first visit to the hospital. I was literally shivering with fear and uncertainty. A thousand questions were buzzing around in my mind as I sat in the waiting room for my turn. My husband held my hand and asked me to calm down. "Everything will turn out well," he said.

After examining me and going through all the investigation reports, the doctor confirmed the diagnosis of Stage 2 breast cancer. I tried to look brave as I sat in the consulting room and masked all emotions, but internally I was weeping. What now? The doctor was very kind, and he reassured me that I could fight this cancer and that he, along with his team, would be with me the whole way. Hearing his words, I started weeping.

First, I underwent some more tests like an ultrasound abdomen and PET CT. These tests are done basically to ensure that cancer has not spread anywhere else. I was lucky that the cancer had not spread and was confined to one lump in the left breast. Now came the treatment planning. It is an ordeal, to be sure. But it is important to be involved in it. It helps you understand what you can expect in the days to come.

Till now, I didn't have a clear understanding of the treatment involved. I vaguely associated terms like chemo and RT with cancer but had no clear idea what they meant.

The medical team explained to me that the treatment would involve three steps: Surgery, Chemotherapy, and Radiation therapy. They told me that the combination of all three gave the best results in terms of cancer cure. I underwent surgery on November 4, 2020. The surgery was successful, and the pathology report after the surgery confirmed that the cancer lump in my breast had been removed completely and the surrounding tissues were clear.

Now it was time for chemotherapy. I had heard about the severe side effects of this treatment. I also knew that there would be hair fall and blackened nails. However, once again, the doctors at KGMU reassured me that all these would be temporary.

They said, "Believe us. You will overcome this." That was literally the day I saw hope and my fight against cancer became easier. Chemotherapy as such did not cause too many side effects like nausea and vomiting because these days, there are medicines to manage them. However, what upset me most was the loss of my hair. It started falling out in clumps two weeks after the first chemo schedule. I started chemotherapy in November 2020 and completed it in March 2021.

My only question to the doctors through this period was when my hair would grow back. My doctor even commented jokingly, "You are more worried about your hair than about your disease." My advice to anyone undergoing chemotherapy is to please invest in a good wig if the loss of hair is upsetting you. It can build your confidence like nothing else can.

A fortnight after my last round of chemo, I started getting radiation therapy. My treatment ended on June 26, 2021. I found strength and courage to face the treatment ordeal in the positive attitude and determination of the entire medical team. They always took the time to listen to my concerns and speak words of encouragement. I breathed a sigh of relief on the final day of radiation therapy. It felt like a burden long-suppressed had finally been let go. I had beaten this thing. The cancer had taken a toll on me physically, emotionally, and financially. But I was cancer-free now. I wanted to celebrate. I have to thank all the doctors and the staff on the medical team, without whose support I would not have reached this day. I am truly grateful for the new lease of life that you have given me. You were dedicated, thoughtful, and compassionate doctors who went beyond the call of duty in working tirelessly for all the patients in your care. I feel blessed to have been under your care, and I greatly appreciate all that you have done for me on this journey of mine. A BIG THANK YOU TO THE ENTIRE TEAM.

My tribute is to all cancer patients, irrespective of what stage you have reached in your personal journey. Maybe you have just received your diagnosis, or you are part way through your treatment, or you have completed your therapy. No matter what, remember you are brave and strong. As you battle cancer and at the same time take care of your families, keep a positive attitude. And be sure to celebrate small victories. I am also thankful to all my family members who stood with me through this arduous journey. My family looked after me and my home. They surrounded me with their love and positivity and prayers. But most of all, I am thankful for my husband, who stood like a rock behind me. He did not let me get scared or demotivated at any time. He fought this cancer along with me. I know this is not the end. I do need to go for regular follow up to ensure that the cancer does not come back. I have to live with the side effects of radiation therapy, like pain in the ribs. However, now I think I can overcome every pain with such a supportive family beside me. And to everyone who is presently on this journey to battle cancer or has already completed their treatment, I say: BE POSITIVE IN YOUR OUTLOOK. NEVER LOSE HOPE. READ UP ABOUT YOUR CANCER. SURROUND YOURSELF WITH POSITIVE PEOPLE.

Remember you are brave and strong.
Do not hesitate to take the help of family and friends. Surround yourself
with positivity.

Azmi's take on her diagnosis is a little different from what Suraiya described. Azmi comes from a more educated background. She works as a teacher. Her world does not only revolve around her home and family. There is a bigger circle to which she belongs professionally.

This definitely has a role in how her diagnosis affected her. She is not so much in despair about how she would be looked at by society. Her fears are more to do with only what she would have to face physically. She mentions she is worried about losing her hair.

Eventually, there are many people who support her in her journey. Her immediate family, extended family, friends, and colleagues all play a role in extending their support, and she gratefully acknowledges and accepts it. Her focus is on celebrating each victory in the fight against cancer. She too ends her story on a note of hope by encouraging cancer survivors never to lose hope. She knows she has to live with the constant follow-up and the side effects of radiation therapy, such as pain in the ribs. Surround yourself with positive people: this statement of hers embodies the universal truth that it is easy to face any difficulty when you have someone standing by you. Cancer affects women from economically privileged as well as economically deprived backgrounds.

However, there may be some differences in how they perceive their disease and the fears and problems they face. Also, there may be differences in the challenges they face as cancer survivors.

Acceptance of the disease for what it is can be seen more among the urban and educated population. At the same time, women from the rural areas and those who are economically weaker have to deal with societal taboos and perceptions to a larger extent. When you are educated and have a job, you really do not worry about what the neighbor thinks of you. But for rural women, their world beyond their immediate family is the social circle, the village, the street, the home. Mastectomy can affect women emotionally as well as physically irrespective of their background. It is important that all women who have undergone mastectomy be offered the choice of breast support, prosthesis, or breast reconstructive surgery.

Addressing this issue can go a long way in making a cancer survivor's life better. It restores their confidence to face society and their worth as a woman.

An article published in *Scroll.in*[23] in December 2021 quotes a postgraduate surgical trainee in the All India Institute of Medical Sciences, Delhi, "Women never bring it up...because the more women speak about it, many more will choose the option of reconstruction." She is talking about women availing themselves of the option of breast reconstruction after a mastectomy. Women usually do not talk about this because either they are not aware of it or they simply do not understand the concept.

In our country, following cancer therapy, women commonly suffer from psychiatric problems, adjustment problems, depression, and anxiety. Much of these symptoms are compounded by the loss of a breast. However, reconstructive surgery can be expensive, and many women may not be able to afford it after already bearing the cost of the cancer treatment. Being declared cancer-free is a time of celebration for anyone, but women who have undergone mastectomy may not be able to truly celebrate. They just accept that it is a consequence of breast cancer and there is nothing they can do about it. The husband or other family members do not truly understand this impact on the woman. They want to focus on cancer and its treatment. They want the woman to become cancer-free. Even when given the option of reconstructive surgery, many women do not opt for it. They feel inhibited to even talk about the option in the presence of the male members of the family. Ignorance about the procedure and fear of increasing the financial burden for the family are two of the main reasons for this. Another reason for women not opting for reconstructive procedures is that most insurance schemes do not cover this. Women need to be made aware of other resources that they can avail themselves of, such as wigs, bra inserts, and padding.

---

[23]https://scroll.in/article/1012212/the-unspoken-scars-of-breast-cancer-survivors-in-india

It is good to become a part of a support group for cancer survivors. These groups can help you deal with your emotions and fears. Support groups usually comprise patients and other breast cancer survivors who lend emotional support to each other. Listening to the journey of a fellow cancer survivor can motivate you to take control of your life. You can start a support group comprising breast cancer survivors. You can organize social meetings and awareness activities in the society and be an ambassador for 'Cure of Cancer.' You will realize that you are not alone, and others, too, are facing similar challenges in their life after cancer. You will be better prepared to handle challenges that come your way. Group therapy is a unique way to come together as a cancer survivor community and lend support to each other.

In rural areas, healthcare workers can arrange these group sessions in sub-centers or primary health centers and encourage all breast cancer survivors from neighboring areas to attend. Women may open up more among their peers about the various issues than they would with a clinical psychologist in a one-on-one session.

Many women find their strength in spirituality and religion. In fact, religious faith would have played an important role in their successful fight against breast cancer. It can continue to help you make the best of your second chance at life. The strength from spirituality can help women welcome positivity and hope into their lives. In summary, each cancer survivor has challenges and concerns, whether they are from rural or urban areas. To cope with these challenges, the first step is to identify and recognize the concerns. Understand what you are facing and talk to your family or friends who support you. Where required, take professional help or counseling. A cancer survivor can find it difficult to get back to normal activity or their usual professional life. All these issues can be faced with the proper support and counseling. Do not hesitate to ask for help. Discuss all health needs, pain, psychological problems, fatigue, etc., with your healthcare team or your doctor, who can guide you to the right resources.

Cancer rehabilitation services play a huge role in getting breast cancer survivors back on their feet. They help you stay as active as possible and allow you to participate actively in family and work. They can help reduce the side effects of cancer and cancer therapy. They can help you remain independent and improve your quality of life.

7

A WORD OF WISDOM

Knowledge is power

In any field, empowerment includes being up to date in the knowledge pertaining to that field. This is true about breast cancer as well. It is important that all women, whether they are from a rural or urban background, should have complete knowledge of breast cancer. And there is no one better to provide this knowledge than someone who has dedicated their professional life to the diagnosis and treatment of breast cancer. In this chapter, I aim to provide a broad view of breast cancer from a doctor's viewpoint.

Breast Cancer Demographics

Breast cancer is the most common cancer that occurs in Indian women, be they from rural or urban areas. It is said to account for 14 percent of all cancers in women. Presently, 1 in 28 women has a lifetime risk of developing breast cancer.

Demographically, it would be 1 in 22 women in the urban areas and 1 in 60 women in the rural areas. Breast cancer accounts for more than 27 percent of all new cancer cases. We are witnessing an increase in the number of cancer patients being diagnosed these days. This absolute increase can be credited to the increase in the population as well as increased access to health facilities. This trend is likely to grow in the coming years. One alarming fact is the drop in the age at diagnosis of breast cancer. Previously, new breast cancer cases were from the age group below 55 years. A majority of the new breast cancer cases are diagnosed in women below 50 years of age. It is clear that younger women are being affected increasingly in the present times. Nearly 50 percent of these women with breast cancer are diagnosed in stage 3, and 15 to 20 percent of women with breast cancer make their first visit to a doctor when the cancer is at stage 4.

We have seen in the previous chapters that breast cancer affects not just the patient, but also the entire family. It extracts an emotional as well as a financial toll on the whole family. The cost of cancer treatment can have far-reaching financial implications for the family. Late detection of breast cancer results in low survival rates. The only way to improve the survival rate is by increasing awareness of the disease among women. Breast cancer is a treatable disease, and the chances of survival are higher when it is diagnosed earlier. Awareness of breast cancer and how it presents, recognizing the early symptoms, and knowing how to perform breast self-examination can help in the early pick up of symptoms.

Causes of Breast Cancer

Breast cancer has been attributed to numerous factors, but the exact cause is still unknown. A number of risk factors for developing breast cancer have been identified and I have elaborated on these in the next chapter. Some of the risk factors include genetics and heredity, sedentary lifestyle, use of oral contraceptive pills, early menarche, late menopause, excessive intake of alcohol, smoking, obesity, and many more.

Basically, these are of two kinds: modifiable risk factors and non-modifiable risk factors. Modifiable risk factors are those that can be avoided, such as obesity. Non-modifiable risk factors are those over which a person does not have any control, such as increasing age, family history, or carrying the *BRCA* gene.

However, many women who have no identifiable risk factors develop breast cancer, while others who are at very high risk do not get affected. Lactation is said to provide some protection to women against breast cancer.

Symptoms of Breast Cancer

I have enumerated the various symptoms associated with breast cancer in another chapter in this book. However, this is important knowledge that cannot be stressed enough, and I enumerate the symptoms that one needs to look out for here as well.

- Change in the size, shape, or appearance of the breast.
- A lump in the breast or the axilla (armpit region).
- Changes in the skin over the breast, such as dimpling.
- Inversion of the nipple.
- Scaling, peeling, or crusting of skin around the nipple.
- Redness in the skin over the breast.
- Blood or any unusual discharge from the nipple.

STAGES OF BREAST CANCER

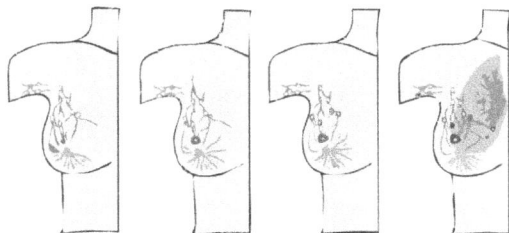

Early Stage   Late Stage

Unique Characteristics Seen in Indian Breast Cancer Patients

Indian patients have some presenting features that are different and unique to this population. They present at a younger age compared to those in Western countries. The average age of presentation in Indians and those in Western nations is 46 years versus 56 years, respectively. Indians present at a more advanced stage of cancer. Indian breast cancer patients also seem to show a higher prevalence of triple-negative cancers.

Treatment Options

There are four treatment methods: surgery, chemotherapy, radiotherapy, and hormonal therapy. Treatment usually involves multiple options. The treatment protocol is formulated based on the type of cancer and the stage of the disease. Most often, patients are initially treated either with surgery or chemotherapy.

Radiotherapy is indicated in selected patients who have undergone breast conservation surgery or patients with advanced-stage breast cancer. Hormone therapy, too, is indicated in a select group of patients whose tumor tissue on pathological examination reveals the presence of hormone receptors. When breast cancer is detected early, breast conservation surgery can be offered to the patient.

Psychologically, this is a better option for the patient than removing the entire breast. In some early-stage breast cancer patients, chemotherapy can be avoided as well.

Role of Biopsy in Diagnosis of Cancer

A biopsy is an investigative procedure that plays a major role in the diagnosis of cancer. Biopsy provides information about the type of cancer and the aggressiveness of the disease. Apart from studying tissue pathology, the biopsy also helps in the identification of various biomarkers.

These biomarkers classify breast cancer into various subtypes, which helps the oncologist decide about the initial form of treatment (surgery or chemotherapy) and the type of chemotherapy drugs to be used. Biomarkers also help in evaluating response to therapy and the prognosis of the patient.

Diagnosis

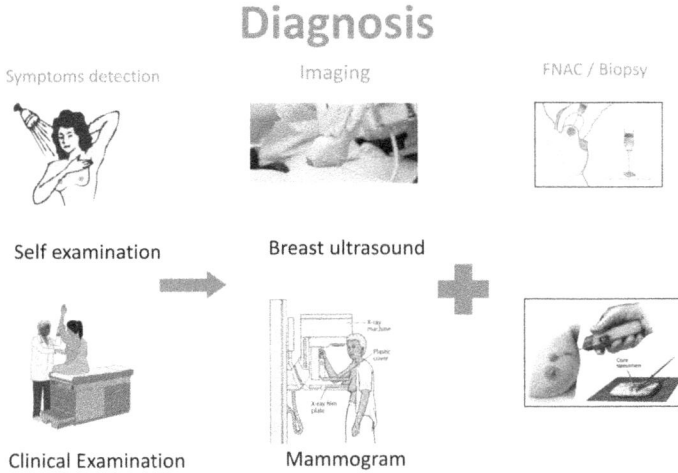

Symptoms detection — Self examination

Imaging — Breast ultrasound

FNAC / Biopsy

Clinical Examination

Mammogram

Adverse Effects on Patient and Family

Breast cancer and its therapy, involving surgery, systemic therapy (chemotherapy, hormonal therapy, targeted therapy, and immunotherapy), and radiation therapy, can adversely affect the physical and mental health of not only the patient but of the other family members as well.

In addition, it affects the quality of life and economic status of the patient and her family. In many instances, there is a fear of recurrence of cancer. This sometimes leads to overtreatment of the condition, thereby increasing the cost of treatment many-fold and taxing the patient and her family financially.

Overtreatment not only increases the financial burden but also places unnecessary physical stress on the patient who has to bear the toxic side effects of cancer therapy.

Cancer Survival Rates

India does not have good survival rates for breast cancer due to the large population, low awareness ratio, presentation at advanced stages, late diagnosis, lack of breast cancer screening programs, lack of appropriate medical facilities, and the high cost of targeted therapies. One out of two women diagnosed with breast cancer die within five years of the diagnosis, which effectively implies a 50 percent mortality rate. Most of the patients in urban areas are diagnosed at stage 2, which is when the lesion becomes a palpable lump.

Challenges in our Healthcare System

In spite of many healthcare measures taken by the various governments, access to quality healthcare remains a challenge to most Indians. Those below the poverty line, daily wage earners, and those living in the numerous villages of India cannot easily afford tertiary healthcare for a disease such as cancer.

The affluent and the educated are aware of breast cancer and the resources at their disposal. The need of the hour is better screening facilities at the grassroots level, creating more awareness about the disease among the people, regular screening programs, easy accessibility to therapy, awareness about the resources that patients and their families can avail themselves, post-treatment support, etc. I have addressed some of these issues in the other chapters in detail.

Social Media—Boon or Bane?

I have found that many patients get the wrong information from online sources. The Internet can be a good resource for information if you access only reputed websites. But how do you identify the reputed websites? The vast majority of our population does not have the awareness to choose the correct source of information online.

Google and social media can, at many times, do more harm than good. I feel that about 30 percent of material found on WhatsApp and other social media constitutes misinformation. This is especially alarming when we specifically talk about cancer. Doctors call this the 'IDIOT Syndrome': 'Internet-derived information obstructing treatment.' It is largely seen in urban areas. Patients read many things on the Internet and get thoroughly confused; this hinders treatment.

One in three articles related to cancer found online or shared through social media has been found to contain elements of misinformation or potentially harmful assertions. We often find promotion of fraudulent treatments for cancer as well. I have come across inaccurate stories and articles regarding breast cancer on various social media sites. More than half of the alleged claims made on the site about the prevention and treatment of breast cancer are wrong.

A 2019 BBC investigation found advertisements for major commercial brands such as Samsung and Heinz displayed alongside misleading and potentially dangerous videos promoting fake breast cancer cures on YouTube. YouTube does carry a lot of quality videos with accurate information about breast cancer as well.

However, an equal number of videos carry inaccurate and misleading information about breast cancer. Unfortunately, patients are drawn to these misleading videos and follow the advice mentioned there. They begin to undergo the wrong treatment, and by the time they realize their mistake, their cancer would have progressed to an advanced stage. Because of believing the misinformation found online, patients lose out on the chance of recovery from cancer; they also pay a heavy price financially.

Fallout of Misinformation About Cancer

Because of misinformation, breast cancer patients refuse to undergo conventional, evidence-based therapies in favor of unproven therapies, which carry a heightened risk of death.

Patients who rely on unproven 'alternative' therapies to treat breast cancer are nearly six times more likely to die from their cancer than those who undergo scientifically proven treatment.

Patients opting for these unproven remedies need to be cautioned about the misinformation present on social media. Many women leave conventional therapy midway and go for these online remedies. There is a pressing need for spreading awareness about the dangers of misinformation.

Experts in Every Nook and Cranny

Traditionally, we are people who source our health-related information from elders and others around us. Health remedies were mainly home cures passed down through the generations. And while there is much to be said in favor of traditional home cures and remedies, these do not auger well in the treatment of breast cancer.

In India, people consider themselves experts on any and every topic. Giving unsolicited advice is almost a national pastime. These advisers are present everywhere. They are especially gung-ho about giving advice on medical issues. They do not hold back from speaking about any illness, cancer included. Very often, they would in no way be connected to the healthcare field. They are neither doctors nor nurses. They may not even be paramedical workers. Not to mention the fact that they have probably never cared for a breast cancer patient either.

Whatever profession people may be from, literate or illiterate, it does not stop them from voicing their opinion and giving their advice. Patients should be careful about their source of advice. They must think rationally and take decisions.

When someone comes forward to give their opinion, we should not hesitate to question their credentials or their experience. We must judge if people are really qualified to give advice on this matter. Even when consulting the healthcare professional, it is advisable to question why a particular treatment is being suggested and ask for supporting evidence.

However, it is not easy to challenge a self-styled expert. It is easier said than done. We can always ask, "What is the basis of your advice?" "Are you an expert on breast cancer or do you have first-hand experience in providing care or treatment to a breast cancer patient?" "Has any member of your immediate family been diagnosed with breast cancer and undergone therapy for the same?" These are some of the questions that one can ask before listening to any advice.

Patients get confused and bewildered when faced with so many opposing opinions and instructions. Many patients stop their regular cancer treatment based on these so-called experts' opinions and go after other treatment methods or 'pathies' that are not scientifically proven.

This leads to the progression of cancer to an advanced stage and decreases the chance of survival. Haphazard medications also do not help and may lead to complications and increased costs.

Alternative Therapies Not Proven in Breast Cancer

Although you may hear of numerous sure-fire remedies in various alternative medical fields, there is no evidence-based proof of a cure from established breast cancer in any of these lines of treatment.

The allopathic system of treatment for breast cancer is evidence-based and has recorded proof of hundreds and thousands of breast cancer patients who have benefitted from it. When we talk about the other 'pathies' of medicine, there is no proof of large-scale trials or experiments.

Following scientific and evidence-based medicine can help breast cancer patients enormously. Especially when diagnosed at the early stages, the chances of remission are very high with allopathic treatment. Other therapies, such as Ayurveda, Homeopathy, Tibetan or Chinese Medicines, and Naturopathy, can help patients as 'Placebo Therapy.' They may help terminally ill patients and can be used in end-of-life care.

Logistics and Family Matters

As we have seen earlier in another chapter, women do not have much say in health matters, especially in rural areas. Lack of family support and hesitancy to consult male doctors are some of the reasons. In addition, there are a lot of cultural factors that come into play when dealing with health matters in women, especially with respect to cancer. Some people believe that cancer is divine punishment for past misdeeds. Lack of transport and over-dependence on male members of the family can be reasons for not seeking early medical help in breast cancer. Women often overlook their health needs due to household commitments. They are programmed to place the family's welfare before their personal care. There may be a delay in the diagnosis of breast cancer also because of a lack of awareness of the disease and reluctance to visit the doctor. In many south Asian countries, and especially in north Indian families, men are considered the head of the family. It is important, therefore, to create awareness about women's health in general and breast cancer in particular among men. Unless the head of the family is aware of breast cancer and the associated issues, the women in that family will never go even for screening for breast cancer, let alone for treatment of the same.

In our society, even educated women are hesitant to discuss matters relating to the breast or their private parts with their husbands, fathers, or brothers. So, it is important that women's health-related messages should be directed toward men to increase their awareness and sensitivity toward these issues. Only when they are aware and sensitized will they be willing to openly discuss these issues. As the men are responsible for the health of their family members, awareness about breast cancer is paramount. Another reason why men need to be educated is that breast cancer can affect men as well. The stagewise progression of breast cancer in men is similar to that in women, and the treatment is the same as well. The only difference is that male breast cancer progresses from early-stage to advanced-stage more rapidly.

Believe Breast Cancer is Curable

A diagnosis of breast cancer usually throws the entire family into profound shock. The word 'cancer' by itself strikes terror in their hearts and they are completely broken on hearing the news. Many people believe it is the end. That should not be the case. Patients need to be educated that breast cancer is curable in these modern times. It should be looked upon just as we would any other non-communicable disease, such as asthma or hypertension, or a communicable disease, such as tuberculosis. These diseases too if not treated can result in death. Many of these non-communicable diseases require lifelong treatment, while breast cancer treatment is long but of a certain duration.

Once cured, you can stop the treatment and live as a normal healthy person. We see that trauma is responsible for so many deaths around us. And in this present era of the pandemic, we have seen so many people who were absolutely healthy lose their lives to Covid-19 in a very short span of time.

The one thing that is certain is the uncertainty of life, and that pertains to cancer as well. Yes, people can lose their lives to cancer just as they do to so many other causes. But early diagnosis and correct and complete treatment can greatly improve survival. Here we have to understand the phrase, "BIOLOGY OF THE CANCER IS KING." This means that 'bad biology' indicates limited survival, even after cancer is cured.

Measures to Tackle Breast Cancer

From a doctor's perspective, I would say that the two most important areas that need to be improved on with regard to breast cancer diagnosis are increasing awareness among people and promoting breast self-examination in women.

We need to come up with strategies by which a greater number of women may be engaged in breast cancer awareness campaigns. I feel that it is important for breast cancer survivors to be made brand ambassadors of awareness campaigns for this disease.

Hearing directly from these survivors will lend confidence and courage to other women suffering from breast cancer so that they too can be cured. Women should be encouraged to practice periodic breast self-examinations.

The need of the hour is to teach women from both rural and urban areas the correct method of performing a breast self-examination. They also need to be encouraged to share their concerns with friends, colleagues, and members of their family. Women should know how their breasts look and feel normally and they should be able to identify any changes and report them to their healthcare provider immediately.

All women above the age of 20 should be encouraged to practice breast self-examination, and women above 40 years of age should be encouraged to undergo periodic screening mammography. The awareness about these measures can be spread in hospitals and other places where women gather.

Survivor Support

Breast cancer survivors face numerous physical and mental challenges. There is not much awareness about this in our society. I think we need to form support groups to address these survivor issues.

There are many support groups functioning in Western countries. We need to form self-help groups and support groups in every region and city for breast cancer survivors. These groups can address the various post-treatment issues faced by these survivors.

The success stories of patients who have completed their treatment serve to increase the confidence of newly diagnosed breast cancer patients and also help those still undergoing treatment to complete their therapy. Support groups have many roles to play.

They not only provide courage and hope, but they also act as guides and help patients in treatment completion. We have a vibrant support group at King George's Medical University, Lucknow, named "Lucknow Breast Cancer Support Group," with the same objectives (www.lbcsg.com).

Common Myths

I have included some common myths regarding breast cancer that I have faced over the years.

- **Myth 1: Breast cancer is not curable.**
  Fact: It is curable if detected early. To be cured of breast cancer, you must undergo scientifically proven investigations and treatment.

- **Myth 2: Breast cancer is contagious or infectious.**
  Fact: It is neither infectious nor contagious.

- **Myth 3: Breast conservation surgery is unsafe compared to a complete mastectomy.**
  Fact: Breast conservation surgery plus radiation therapy is as safe as a complete mastectomy. However, the decision is usually made by the oncologist after taking into consideration the stage and grade of the tumor.

- **Myth 4: All breast lumps are cancers.**
  Fact: It must be remembered that all lumps that appear in the female breast are not cancerous in origin. There are enough sophisticated investigative techniques these days to differentiate a malignant (cancerous) tumor from a benign (non-cancerous) one. In general, breast lumps that occur in the young are not malignant, and a lump that appears after 40 years of age should be considered malignant until proved otherwise by investigations.

- **Myth 5: Men cannot get breast cancer.**

Fact: Breast cancer is rare in men, but they do get it. About one percent of breast cancer patients are men.

- **Myth 6: Breast cancer always presents with a lump either in the breasts or in the armpit (axilla).**

Fact: It is true that the most common symptom of breast cancer is a painless lump in the breasts or the axilla; however, that is not the only symptom. Breast cancer can also present as nipple deviation, nipple retraction, ulceration of the nipple, or discharge from the nipple with or without a lump. It may also present as a change in the shape or feel of the breast, skin thickening, ulceration, and orange peel-like appearance of the skin of the breast.

- **Myth 7: Breast cancer is an old woman's disease.**

Fact: As per data for the year 2020, 1.78 lakh new cases of breast cancer were diagnosed in India. Out of these, 1.32 lakh patients were above the age of 40 and the rest were below 40. Breast cancer in young patients has comparatively more aggressive clinical and biological characteristics and a less favorable outcome compared to that of breast cancer in older patients. Breast cancer awareness among youngsters is the need of the hour to reduce its mortality and morbidity.

⚜

SURVIVOR NOTES

Name: Neetu Rastogi
Age: Undisclosed
Location: Lucknow

People often say ignorance is bliss. The lesser one knows, the better it is. But is this always true? I am a woman, married to a wonderful man, and the mother of two beautiful children. I ran my household with a smile on my face always; life was good.

I was doing well. I was happy and my family was happy. We had nothing much to worry about. But my destiny had scripted a new story for the year 2016!

It was my birthday, March 9, 2016. It was a beautiful day and I was very happy. Many of my childhood friends called to wish me. Long phone calls, chatting, and reliving the golden days of childhood—everything seemed blissful that day. I was so engrossed in that joy that I had almost forgotten about the knotted nodule I had felt earlier in my breast. As they say, childhood friends can take away all your pain. I too was basking in the memories, utterly ignorant of the looming dark clouds of worries.

The day waned by, and my husband casually enquired about the lump. I checked and found it was still knotted at the same place.

"I think we should consult a doctor. It's not usual." He suggested we go to my regular doctor. A distressing thought crossed my mind—could it be cancer? As the doctor asked about my concerns, I informed her that I had felt a lump in my breast that didn't disappear even after the monthly cycle was over. She looked concerned and checked me physically. "I think we should get a mammography done."

I had heard the word 'breast cancer'; I had seen posters in hospitals and diagnostic centers.

But, as I mentioned at the beginning, ignorance is sometimes a kind friend. Until we fall into the pit, we don't look carefully at the road. I was petrified. I underwent X-ray mammography, and it was then I discovered this new, unimagined script that was written for my life. The doctor suggested that I undergo further testing, specifically an FNAC, to confirm the diagnosis. Back home, I found it impossible to sleep with all that medical jargon hovering inside my head. It took a day to get all my test reports in hand. My husband looked worried seeing them but wouldn't tell me anything despite repeated inquiries. Something was indeed alarming! I hardly slept a wink that night.

The dawn of March 11, 2016, was tainted with the smell of fear. I didn't even go for my usual morning walk. I felt as if I was getting lost in the darkest alley of life. I never harmed anyone; why was I suffering? Who would take care of my two sons once I was gone? I had heard that cancer treatment was quite expensive. Where would we get the money from? My elder son was pursuing hotel management at IHM, Goa, and the younger one was studying in the 8th standard. We had saved money for the children's future; how could I use it for my treatment? Probably, I had only a few months to survive and God wished to take me closer to him. Nothing seemed to be working. How could I contract this disease? Did I eat anything wrong? I was not even aware of how it spread.

Today, if I sit and summarize my life, I would say, *"Jaanko Raakhe Saaiyan, Maar Sakhe Na Koi!"* (One who is under the guidance of God, cannot be harmed.) My father's friend's son was the HOD of the Radiation Oncology department at Dr. Ram Manohar Lohiya Hospital. My husband and my brother went to him with my reports. He advised getting operated on immediately to eliminate the tumor and then proceeding with the other treatment. Now the next question was whom to go to for the operation. He suggested that we meet Dr. Anand Kumar Mishra. The doctor used to attend the OPD on Mondays and Thursdays. Monday was already gone, but we got an appointment for Tuesday. We met with the doctor at his office in KGMU.

He, too, was of the opinion that immediate surgery was required. "Do you wish to remove the breast?" The doctor asked for our opinion. How could we say anything? We had nothing to opine or decide when my life was at stake. My husband and I unanimously requested the doctor to take a suitable call. Back home, I was haunted by my fears. Who would take care of the household if I was gone? Worried and confused, I asked my housemaid to help me get someone trustworthy for cooking and washing the clothes. Suddenly, everything seemed to be falling in place. God seemed to be helping me in making arrangements. My treatment was to begin the next day. Now, I could relax and go for my treatment.

However, the main hiccup was what to tell my parents. They wouldn't be able to accept such news. Thinking it over, I decided to tell them I was having a simple operation for a nodule in the breast. But as parents, they were worried, no matter what. To date, their words keep ringing in my ears: God will take care of everything. If he has inflicted the pain, he himself will get you out of it.

After the necessary tests, my operation was scheduled for March 21, 2016. I got an earlier schedule for my operation as the festival of Holi was approaching in the next two days. I was admitted to KGMU on March 19, 2016. My stomach quaked as I was made to lie on the operation table. Worried and anxious, I wasn't sure of anything. Just before giving anesthesia, I was asked which breast was to be operated on: right or left? The ward assistant inquired and started preparing my operation site. My operation went on for four hours, and the doctors did a posture corrective surgery for my right breast too. I am just a common person with mediocre intellect, and I was amazed that these skilled surgeons could perform even the unplanned surgery successfully. Somehow, destiny seemed to be favoring me. I found myself in the ward when I regained consciousness. Notwithstanding the blurred vision and my still stuck, drowsy eyelids, I could figure out a nurse sitting by my side. I inquired about my family and she agreed to call them in. I was soon shifted to a private room. I had read somewhere that if one keeps walking after the operation, one heals quickly. I had to get well soon.

My younger son's final exams were approaching and I had to sit with him during his lessons. My motherly instincts couldn't relax even amidst the lofty walls of the hospital. I was discharged after two days and was again called for a check-up after seven days. I presumed that once the operation was done, everything was fine. I never knew that the actual battle was going to begin now.

As the saying goes, if the beginning is good, the end is bound to be good too. The doctors at KGMU had set the beginning of my battle with cancer on a good note by doing a successful operation.

I went with my husband to the radiotherapy department of another government hospital in Lucknow to schedule my radiotherapy sessions. The doctor there asked me not to get bogged down with the problems that come along with the treatment.

"You have to settle the lives of your children. If you give up, who will take care of them?" At that moment, I failed to comprehend the gravity of his words. The course of treatment was long. I had to undergo eight sessions of chemotherapy, followed by 20 sessions of radiation therapy. Once they were over, I had to undergo hormone therapy for a year. The disease itself was scarring enough and now the treatment regime was scaring me.

My first session of chemotherapy began on April 14, 2016. I got admitted to the ward. There was a time when I was so scared of needles/injections, but now with so many tests being performed so often, I had lost count of the number of pricks. The first attempt at placing the intravenous (i.v.) canula resulted in a ruptured vein with excessive bleeding. After multiple attempts, the medical staff finally got my i.v. going. The chemotherapy session was a long one, lasting from 11.00 in the morning till 5.00 in the evening. I felt dizzy and nauseous. My husband brought me some tea but I had to decline. When I finally reached home, I was drained of all energy. After a bath, I stretched out on my bed with a sigh. There was a constant urge to vomit and pass motion. I anxiously awaited the arrival of the dawn, hoping it would bring me some relief. The night seemed to stretch on as if it would never end.

The next morning, I met the doctor again. I had not eaten anything the previous night nor that morning. I had felt a stabbing pain in my throat and couldn't eat anything then either. The doctor prescribed some medicines and asked me to rest well. I developed ulcers in my throat, and I noticed that I was beginning to lose my hair in a couple of weeks. I had been advised to get a blood test done after 15 days. I could neither eat nor drink anything and was almost bedridden.

I had lost all interest in food because of those ulcers in my mouth and throat. It was difficult to even drink water. I lay like a soulless body. Any disease is a challenge; however, the diagnosis of cancer instills a distinct threat to the entire family. It not only causes immense physical distress to the patient but also causes a lot of emotional turmoil in those around. My worsening condition scared my younger son. He often asked his father if I would ever get well, if I would be normal like before. I felt an emptiness welling up in me as my fears intensified. What if I were to die? How will my children cope?

My elder son was in Goa at that time, pursuing his hotel management course. I hadn't informed him about my cancer, lest he should be worried. I never made any video call to him. He seemed to sense that something was amiss and asked me once if I was not keeping well, and why my voice sounded different. I never disclosed anything to him. However, I often mulled over these thoughts. If I never recovered, I wouldn't be able to see my children. For a mother, it was indeed a stressful thought. My husband often tried to convince me that I would be alright and would soon get back to my usual routine. But, somehow, my mind was not ready to accept that. I was emotionally torn to an extent beyond recovery.

It is only during the difficult phases in life that we get to see the faces of people beyond the masks they wear and discern between true and forged concern. I lived in a joint family: My husband and I lived with my husband's parents and his elder brother's family, which included his wife and their two kids.

I was overwhelmed by the support they provided. My mother-in-law never let me miss my mother. She used to feed me with fruits or a bowl of lentils, just as my own mother would do. She took care of the whole household. She put up a brave façade and used to say that I had to get alright quickly to help them in their old age. She always tried to motivate me but often shed tears in front of my husband. She was concerned that the family would be shattered if anything ever happened to me. My in-laws were entirely dependent on me for the household chores and she worried about their old age. I was more of a daughter than a daughter-in-law to them.

Many relatives used to come home to see me. Everyone wished to know about how I was coping with the treatment. It often made me think that I wouldn't survive long. It was quite uncomfortable to talk about my ailment all the time. I was always feeling low and used to bicker with almost everyone. I never realized what had actually happened to me. I used to shout at anything spoken out of order.

Fifteen days later, the blood report showed a lowered total leukocyte count and red blood cell count. I was prescribed some injections to increase the blood count; unless the blood count increased, I couldn't receive the next round of chemotherapy on the twenty-first day. I developed some reddening in the abdomen and numbness in my legs after my first chemo. I was experiencing spasms of pain as well. My nails turned dark and hard. It was difficult to breathe or sit up for a long time. There was loss of bladder control as well. There were wounds in my legs too. The doctor explained that these were side effects of chemotherapy. Sometimes I sat and wondered how far that small knot in my breast had brought me. Every part of my body was now weak with some problem or the other. My second chemo was scheduled for May 7, 2016. I was emotionally exhausted. No matter how much my husband tried to convince me, I was adamant about not wanting to undergo any more chemotherapy. I spent the whole night weeping. I dreaded looking at myself in the mirror. Every scrap of normalcy was snatched from me.

Fear of losing my husband and my family constantly lingered within me. Half the time, I didn't know which part of my body was giving me trouble as the pain was all-pervasive. I was sleep-deprived, and I sought only one promise from my husband with my tear-soaked eyes. I could bear any kind of treatment only if he remained by my side. He hugged me tight, cupped my face, and promised to be with me forever, come what may.

With the second chemo over, my eyes kept a watch on the clock. I was pondering about the next six sessions I had to undergo. Each chemo usually lasted for six to seven hours. I felt hapless and hopeless. I could neither eat nor sleep properly. I just used to close my eyes and lie on the cot. A woman is supposed to be the epitome of patience; however, mine had gone for a toss. I was irritated all the time. I didn't like to eat or sleep or talk or anything. Everyone tried to persuade me to eat. I had to gain some strength as the doctors would stop the treatment if the hemoglobin levels fell.

The more I looked at the mound of tablets, the more I was maddened. It seemed only these tablets were my food. My mouth and throat were filled with ulcers. Only a few strands of hair were left on my head. The wounds on the legs were deep and that numbness still persisted. My nose picked up a peculiar stench from every kind of food. I could withstand only citrus fruits and lentils. I developed a weird kind of aversion toward *rotis* but still had to eat them. Though reluctant toward eating, I continued taking dates, sprouts, green tea, and green vegetables regularly with the hope of getting healed soon.

It seemed my problems were not going to end any time soon. My bleeding continued and I couldn't control my bladder. I didn't have much sensation in my legs. I was unable to walk without any support. I tried but was always worried about falling down.

My days were an unending cycle of trips to the hospital and back home. I often wondered if my remaining life was going to be spent in such regular hospital visits. Between two sessions of chemo, I was spending almost 10 days on the hospital premises. Chemotherapy added the problem of piles too.

Even with Cremaffin laxative, it was still difficult to pass motion. With so many unwarranted issues cropping up, there were times when I felt death was a better option. I was thoroughly depressed and used to cry the whole day. One day my mother said, "If you get bogged down like this, how can your father and I survive? You are our strength. Read out the 11th and 18th chapters of Bhagavad Geeta. It will impart some emotional strength."

Her words brought some change to my mindset. Instead of lying on the cot and scrutinizing the 'why me' attitude, reading the Geeta would be a sort of change. I decided to follow her advice.

The Bhagavad Geeta says thus: *There is always a reason behind every bad thing that happens to us. It is possible that you are a pious soul but God wishes to cleanse you from any kind of sin and that's why he is inflicting pain. Who knows you were entitled to a worse situation but God culminated your ill fate on a smaller scale.*

I was moved by these words. I started devoting some time to worshipping God; not only because I had to beg for my life, but to stop myself from being bedridden. Honestly, there was a drastic shift in my thinking process. I gradually nurtured a bit of optimism. I started having a proper breakfast and switched to foods that would improve my hemoglobin level. Soon, the third and fourth chemo sessions were over. I was now habituated to all the consequences. I accepted the troubles and decided to move on with the treatment.

Many relatives called and shared their opinion during my treatment. Someone suggested that I go visit a *Vaidya* in Varanasi. He seemed to have a permanent cure for cancer. Someone's cousin got treated there, they said. One of the relatives advised me to go for homeopathy treatment, which didn't have so many side effects, while others opined for Ayurveda in Kerala. I was asked to shift to Kerala and get treated there itself. Some thought it would be better to get treatment in a big city such as Delhi or Mumbai; people suggested that I visit another private cancer institute instead of remaining in Lucknow. However, my husband and I decided to complete the course of allopathic treatment first and then decide on other alternatives. My paternal aunt and her husband were doctors.

They advised me to get treated locally because I could meet the doctors as and when required. That comfort would not be possible if I went to a different city for the treatment. I had known people losing their beauty after a terrible accident or as they grew old. I could never believe that a treatment procedure could bring such a terrible change in my looks. I hardly recognized myself in the mirror. Not a single strand of hair stood on my scalp. Everyone said that once the chemo was over, I would get back my hair. However, as I ran my fingers on my scalp, I wasn't convinced. I was hesitant to go in front of people. On the same note, I didn't cover my head inside the premises of my home.

My hair used to fall in clumps and would be scattered throughout the house. Be it in the bedroom or the bathroom, over the bed or the pillows, it was hair everywhere. Sometimes I wished that I would lose all my hair at once and not in fits and starts. Covering my head with a stole constantly reminded me of my lost hair and that impacted my confidence very much. When I completed my third and fourth sessions of chemo, I realized that pain and depression had become my closest companions. My weight had gone down to 45 kilograms and I was looking more like a bundle of bones. Nothing or no one could liberate me from these rusted shackles of cancer.

My radiation sessions started on July 12, 2016. One can fathom the convolution of cancer when one finds every cancer survivor remembering their dates of treatment. Diseases can kill; however, in the case of cancer, the patient is slowly crippled by the side effects. Within two to three sessions of radiation therapy, I developed a wound in the breast, oozing out a watery fluid. Doctors said that everything would be fine once the radiation was over. They advised to clean the wound with Betadine and keep it covered with a cotton pad. My repeated visits to the hospital heartened me that I was not alone. There were so many people around with much more difficult and baffling conditions. Patients who had undergone surgery and chemotherapy in Delhi, Mumbai, and Allahabad were now queued up here in the radiation department for radiotherapy.

There was a cancer patient at every corner trying to give a tough fight against the disease. Patients with oral and throat cancers were difficult to look at. Their faces were distorted and they could hardly speak. I could see them miming. Something whispered that I was actually in a better state with breast cancer. I had lost my hair and my beauty, but my face wasn't misshapen. I could talk to my loved ones. I could see my breast color changing during the radiation. The radiation rays burned the skin. Bathing was prohibited during the course of radiation as water accumulation on the radiation spot could lead to sores.

By August 5, 2016, the course of 20 radiation cycles was completed. It was followed by four sessions of chemo again. And it was then that I developed a few more problems. I got wounds in every sensitive part of my body and it was difficult to sit or stand. The skin specialist confirmed it as a fungal infection that was a side effect of the present chemo medicine. My legs still had numbness, and sometimes I doubted if I would ever get back the normal sensation in my legs. My hands would pain even when I wore the lightest bangles. Toe-rings caused wounds. I always felt nauseated, and honestly, by now I was quite used to these ulcers in my mouth and throat.

Gradually, my body got used to the chemotherapy drugs, but the fungal infection persisted. The doctor confirmed that the fungal infection would remain till the last dose of Paclitaxel chemotherapy. People add feathers of success to their hats, and here I was getting thorns of symptoms poking my head with every session of chemo!

As per the treatment regime, I had to undergo echocardiography periodically to check on the functioning of my heart. This was because the chemo drugs could affect the heart as well. My heart was found to be functioning at 70 percent, which was acceptable for the continuation of the cancer treatment. Months passed by and finally, my eighth chemo was also over. I sighed a sense of relief as everything was slowly coming on track. Now, I was to begin hormone therapy.

One of the greatest qualities of a good doctor is his/her ability to inject positive vibes into the patient. The chemo and radiation doctor did the same for me. His words were so reassuring. He said, "Half of your treatment is over. You have already won half the battle. All these troubles are trivial before the life ahead. Roam around. Eat well and be happy. You won't even realize how swiftly everything will be over."

True, before I could realize the time, my hormone therapy was completed as well. All these years, the hospital had become my second home. Fifteen days a month, I had to visit the hospital for some reason or the other. Be it for a blood test or ultrasound, X-ray, bone scan, or a routine check-up, going to the hospital was set as the new routine of my life.

The journey of my hormone therapy was a little heart-wrenching. Two of my fellow patients lost their battle against cancer. The irony was, I never found them bogged down. While I witnessed their loss, I discerned the power of the Almighty.

Doctors can provide you with the best of treatments; your grit can be indomitable, yet everything lies in the hands of God. We, humans, are mere players performing according to His plans. My memories shall always hold Savitri Devi and Bhagirathi Devi in a special corner of my heart.

Savitri was from a village near Rai-Bareilly. She was suffering from uterus cancer. Her uterus was removed, but she continued to have pain in the abdomen. She was admitted to the hospital during my second hormone therapy. I found the nurse administering glucose after her second operation.

As I was told, her lungs were filled with water which had spread to the abdomen. The water had to be removed through an operation. She had trouble breathing as well.

Savitri Devi looked like a mere skeleton during my third cycle of hormone therapy. She used to wail in pain and had lost control of her bladder. She passed away due to multiple organ failure during my fourth hormone therapy. I was saddened to the core, as if someone close to my heart had left.

During the whole course of my treatment, I seemed to develop some sort of connection with whomever I met. They all seemed my own. They all were facing the same kind of trauma as I. I couldn't do anything more than just pray for all of them. So much pain around pierced through me.

Bhagirathi Devi was from Guna. She had throat cancer and used to talk in sign language. She couldn't speak. She was doing well after her first dose of chemo but somehow developed a blood clot in the brain and eventually got paralyzed. I was petrified. Muddled, I often asked my husband if I could discontinue my treatment. As a mother of two, I couldn't bear to think that I might leave my children without a mother. However, throughout the process, my husband consoled me to remain positive. My reports were encouraging. I had nothing to worry about.

My husband supported me throughout the treatment: taking me to the hospital, cleaning my room, taking care of my medicines, taking care of the children, and so much more. Not only that, he never uttered a single word about my treatment costs. He always said, "Money will come and go. You just get alright first." His words made me overlook the troubles and proceed with the treatment. No matter how rudely I had spoken, he never took it to heart. He always looked after my needs. As I revisit those days, I realize how husbands never show their true love for their wives openly. But it shines through in their service such as this.

I completed my treatment on September 22, 2017. The doctor prescribed tamoxifen tablets for five years and asked me to come for a routine check-up periodically. He said that it would take two and a half to three years to get back to my normal life. Gradually my bowel movements became smooth. My energy level increased and I could cook on my own. I could even help my kid in his studies.

Life slowly drifted toward normalcy. I was regular with my exercises. I started doing *pranayama* and also went for walks. Even today, I exercise regularly, and I am leading a normal life. The biggest lesson I learned from my disease: Life is full of ups and downs; never lose courage and keep moving.

Cancer treatment is long, and sometimes it seems unending. The side effects are indeed cumbersome. However, as I realized, our mind has a bigger role to play while accepting the treatment. The battle against cancer is not only physical but also mental.

Not only is your body fighting the disease, but your emotions are doing so as well! Cancer treatment needs a mind of steel that is brimfull of positivity, an undying urge to get well soon, and above all, God's blessings.

Lastly, in this crisis of mine, all my relations, whether personal or social, have supported me immensely. The contributions of those angelic doctors and their associates who helped me to recover from such a dreadful disease shall remain unforgettable till I breathe my last. They initiated my treatment with a successful operation. I show my humble gratitude toward my family and all those excellent doctors who helped me in getting this new life.

In the end, it is never dying that scares us. It is always the pain of losing our loved ones. I had an army of friends and family to take care of my children; but still, I grieved for the pain of losing on time. I used to cry until my eyes ran dry and my chest heaved violently.

I kept asking the question, "Why me? Why my children? What wrong had I done?" I know, we all live in a mortal plane. We all will die someday. Still, once in a while, as we spend hours cooking the best of meals for our family, we women must acknowledge our mere existence.

Our health matters. We must not be ignorant about our bodies. Just like our family, our body needs our time, our consideration. I would guess that half the women are not even aware of the symptoms of breast cancer.

Tell me, how many of us check on our breasts or our other private parts? We wake up to fulfill our duties toward our family.

That's the routine of our lives. With my horrendous experience, I would like to urge every woman to be aware of cancer and its symptoms.

Have faith: in God, in your doctor, in your body's ability to heal.
Life is full of ups and downs; never lose courage and keep moving.

Numerous women pass through the portals of King George's Medical University, Lucknow, where I have been working for many years now. I have treated breast cancer patients in different stages of cancer. There have been so many different outcomes. But one thing that I can vouch for is the importance of early diagnosis.

Neetu Rastogi was not really aware of the symptoms of cancer, but she did happen to discover the lump in her breast. She was fortunate that she could approach her husband, who again was aware to some extent of the urgency that the situation merited. When you read the account of her tryst with breast cancer, the reality faced by many women is clear.

The treatment is not easy to bear. The side effects can be demoralizing in the extreme. And there are well-meaning but ignorant friends and relatives urging you to give up on the established treatment regimen and go after fabled therapies that promise an easy cure.

Neetu is from an educated background, with many of her relatives in the medical profession. Even though she pleaded to end the treatment when her suffering was too much for her to bear, her family was extremely supportive and encouraging. They ensured that she was able to complete her treatment. She was fortunate that her entire family stood by her.

Each patient is different. And each patient's experience will be different. Not everyone experiences the same intensity of side effects with chemotherapy and radiation therapy.

Many patients sail through these sessions quite well. It is important not to go by tales told by different well-wishers, but to seek medical help if you suspect that you have a lump in your breast.

The most important requirement in this fight against cancer is the indomitable will to win over the disease and survive. I salute each and every breast cancer patient who has fought the odds successfully and is alive to tell their story.

Name: Kanchan Rawat
Age: 40
Location: Lucknow

We Indians often bask in the preconceived notion that government Hospitals are not good. They neither have good doctors nor the best of facilities, we say. I have even heard people calling government hospitals the stepping stones to mortuaries. Today, as I write about my experience as a breast cancer survivor, I urge people to stop putting down government doctors and doctor hopping. Government hospitals are indeed good and have genuine doctors who do their best to help their patients. I was diagnosed with breast cancer and underwent a mastectomy at one of the prestigious medical college hospitals in India, and I assure you that I was treated by the best of doctors and received the best of treatment.

To begin with, my name is Kanchan Rawat. I am 40 years old, married, and a mother of two. My son is 13 and my daughter is 11. My husband works as a teacher. I was happy in my close-knit family and was enjoying every ounce of familial joy. I had no reason to shed tears—no financial worries or health worries. Life was indeed balanced. And then, suddenly one day, my life was turned upside down and I was pulled into a bottomless pit of despair. My faith in my fate was altered in a fraction of a day. I was pinned down by a disease that no human would ever imagine having. The worst part of my cancer was its abrupt arrival.

When I relive the sequence of events, I realize how ignorant I have been of my health. It was in April 2018 that I first sensed a kind of nodule forming in my right breast. However, I had already planned to visit my parents at Kotdwar and I did not wish to interfere with that. I decided to come back and then pay a visit to my family doctor.

I was not having any pain or discomfort; so, it did not bother me much. Moreover, my parents lived quite far away from me. I could visit them only once or twice a year, so I did not wish to change my plans at all. At that point in time, parents were more important than a mere lump in the breast. I returned in June and then thought of consulting a doctor. One of my sisters, Deveshwari, worked as a staff nurse at King George's Medical University (KGMU). She advised me to go for a consultation in the surgery division of the medical college. I went the very next day, and the doctor advised me to undergo ultrasonography and mammography. The latter did not provide much information and thus I was advised to undergo a biopsy. My maternal uncle worked in the pathology department of KGMU. I immediately sought his guidance and he helped me to get my biopsy done. The report came within ten days only to snatch all peace from my whole life. I was suddenly bereft of my sanity. I could not gauge anything that was happening to me. I could see, but could not find anything good. I could hear but failed to understand any of that medical jargon. Holding that biopsy report, I felt like a shard of glass was tearing through my soul. I was completely broken. However, my uncle, husband, and family stood by my side and rekindled my hope.

I was diagnosed with grade II breast cancer and was advised to go for immediate treatment. However, I was muddled over where to go. I sent the reports to my brother who was residing in Delhi. He consulted some of the specialists in Gangaram Hospital and Apollo Hospital, who suggested that I have my treatment right here at KGMU. Somehow, I was still not convinced. I wished to have a second consultation at the Post Graduate Institute (PGI), Lucknow. My brother-in-law was working in PGI; nevertheless, he too opined for KGMU only. He was dead against my going for treatment to any of the private hospitals and referred me to Dr. Anand Mishra at KGMU. He had been in close association with Dr. Mishra and had already discussed my case with him. Everyone was in favor of KGMU.

But here I was, still coiled up in my own uncertainty. I harbored a weird fear of going to a government hospital. But, as time passed by, my prejudices were washed away. And everyone in my family and friends circle held me tight with their good wishes and positive vibes. I slowly drifted to a positive faith that I would get alright soon. I went to KGMU for a consultation on July 12, 2018.

I got admitted and my operation was scheduled for July 16. Every doubt of mine was cleared as the doctor explained to me the procedures involved. I was now confident that I had come to the correct place for my treatment. Nothing could go wrong where the doctors were not only really friendly and approachable, but also knowledgeable and focused on their roles.

My chemotherapy sessions started 21 days after the surgery. I was terrified, of course. I worried about the hair loss and how I would go anywhere with a bald head. More than the disease, the side effects of the treatment looked dreadful. Also, so much misinformation and rumors were offered to me before my chemotherapy started. Some stated that the drugs were made out of snake poison and worse. For a moment, it took my breath away; however, I soon realized that my aim was to get well, and I should not be unduly bothered about the composition of the medicines. By now, I had absolute trust in the doctors treating me, and I believed they were competent enough to cure my ailment. Everyone in the family and the hospital staff buttressed my morale. They all reassured me that my hair would grow back once the treatment was completed. I received my first chemotherapy on August 7.

I had never seen any chemo patients before. I was a little shaken, but my family stood beside me like a strong pillar of emotional support. My father-in-law took care of me more like a father. Every member of my family prayed along and supported me in this tedious journey of breast cancer treatment. During the course of my treatment, I had witnessed patients who were in a more pitiable state than I was. I was at least able to eat while some were completely bedridden, smitten to almost death. Still, I would say there is more misconception about chemotherapy than facts.

Yes, it can be a painful procedure. But if one decides to get alright, the treatment regime goes on smoothly. The whole endocrine surgery department was extremely supportive. The doctors, nursing staff, and ward boys used to motivate all the patients to think positively. They always reassured every patient about the cure. However, there were so many other people busy pointing out the flaws and pitfalls. Many talked about the untimely death of other cancer patients. In due course of time, I realized that life comes with both good and bad experiences. The only way to attract the good toward you is to think about and focus on the good alone. My experience with cancer affirmed my faith in God and destiny. None can overpower or change what has been already decreed or written by the Almighty. We humans must move on with whatever is served to us. I could overcome those eight sessions of chemotherapy because of my husband's constant support.

I had reduced my interaction with people too and concentrated on my health. By February 15, my radiation therapy started. I had to undergo 24 sessions of radiation, and gradually I could sense the betterment in my body. These days, I am leading a healthy and normal life. I won the gruesome battle with cancer and have completely recovered. With my experience, I would urge every other cancer fighter to develop this fighting spirit. There is nothing to fear. The more you fear, the more you have to lose. Cancer paves a battlefield and we have to fight and not surrender. I am thoroughly indebted to the whole staff at KGMU who took immense care of me and my ailment. I was provided with every kind of support. They are the reason behind my existence today. I could sit and laugh and eat with my loved ones because of the KGMU doctors and nursing staff. As I retrospect, I find myself in a far better situation than what many of those other patients are in. To be honest, my diagnosis did shatter me. I used to curse myself for my past deeds to have got such a dreadful disease. But then, God had sent me so many angelic souls to help me in this battle of mine. I would say 'God' inflicted the problem and provided the solution too. I consider myself luckier than many other people out there.

My husband never let me get bogged down. My uncle helped with my treatment procedures in every way possible. I shall always be indebted to my brother-in-law, Dhan Singh Rawat. He always kept in touch with the doctors and kept abreast of my treatment with regular updates; he kept my morale high. My co-sister and my sister-in-law, Neelam, treated me better than they would a sister. They took care of my family like their own and never let me worry about any of my responsibilities. I can never forget the contributions of Geeta Negi during this darkest phase of my life. In today's world, even your own blood cannot help you like how Geeta *Ji* did for me.

My in-laws took care of me like my own parents. At the brink of 70, they managed the whole household and let me rest. Apart from my own family, I was blessed with so many unrelated souls who helped me emotionally more than anything else. I was always injected with positive thinking. Can I ever forget them? I found angels in the guise of the doctors in the endocrine surgery department at KGMU. The whole course of treatment eliminated my doubts about the facilities in government hospitals. I did initially hop between doctors and hospitals in pursuit of better treatment as I could never believe the availability of competent and able guidance in the crowded corridors of a medical college. KGMU came into my consideration only when my brother-in-law insisted on consulting Dr. Mishra. The ambiance within the hospital and during the treatment was beyond my expectations.

Not a single day did I feel ignored or left out in the milling queue of patients. I am in dearth of words to describe the magnanimity of the doctors who did my radiation therapy. Helpful and considerate, they never allowed me to think of anything other than getting completely healed. I am grateful to each and every soul who held my hands tight and helped me overcome this disastrous disease. And before I conclude, I wish to unveil a wonderful side of Dr. Anand Mishra. Apart from his professional acumen, he is a soul par excellence. His undying endeavor to educate people about breast cancer is incomparable.

Apart from being a great doctor, he is a great human being who is constantly working toward the social welfare of cancer patients. His efforts and contribution deserve a grand salute. As I tread on a new life, I would like to extend my help in his virtuous pursuit toward the betterment of our society. *Government hospitals and the doctors who work there are doing yeomen service. Every cancer fighter has to develop this fighting spirit. There is nothing to fear. The more you fear, the more you have to lose. Cancer paves a battlefield and we have to fight and not surrender.*

We all like stories with happy endings, and for me, there is nothing that makes me happier than to hear the story of a survivor, a breast cancer survivor. The common misconception among the people is that government hospitals are not equipped to handle breast cancer cases. Or people might think that the doctors are not as qualified as those working in corporate or private hospitals. Kanchan's story negates this idea. She begins by saying that this whole preconceived notion of government hospitals not being good or not having adequate facilities should be corrected. She underwent her entire cancer therapy at a government hospital and received the best treatment. Her experience brings a ray of hope to the many women who are pondering where to go for treatment once their cancer has been diagnosed.

Let me assure you that government tertiary care centers have very good facilities and dedicated faculty. The important thing is to begin the treatment as soon as possible and not delay it. Kanchan had picked up her symptom of breast lump early in the course of the disease. This ensures a better chance of complete cure. Kanchan describes the importance of having faith in God and facing challenges with a positive attitude. Yes, a positive attitude can help overcome many of the difficulties that one faces during the treatment. I have seen many women facing their treatment with grit and determination and eventually successfully completing the therapy.

Do not hesitate to take the help of family and friends. You need all the help you can get to face this. There are no guarantees in life, but choosing the right treatment is a step toward recovery.

With perseverance and willpower, I can say a breast cancer patient can indeed beat the odds. Who is likely to develop breast cancer? Is there a sure way to know? In the next chapter, I have discussed some of the risk factors for developing breast cancer in detail.

8

ROLE OF FAMILY HISTORY AND GENETIC FACTORS

Are you at risk of developing breast cancer?

One question that I get asked very often in my profession is this: "Doctor, why did I get breast cancer?" Awareness of the risk factors for breast cancer is very low in our population. Awareness about the role of family history in developing breast cancer is also very poor. Women just know that breast cancer is not a good disease to have and prefer not to think beyond that.

Only when a woman is diagnosed to have breast cancer do the questions arise. Being diagnosed with breast cancer is truly a life-changing moment.

The news can be very difficult to handle at first. Each person's journey is unique in this respect. Cynthia Nixon is an American actress who is a breast cancer survivor. Her mother had breast cancer as well.

This is what she has to say:

Cancer is really hard to go through and it's really hard to watch someone you love go through, and I know because I have been on both sides of the equation.

So, what are the odds that you are likely to get breast cancer if your mother or sister had it? Overall, only five to ten percent of breast cancers are thought to have a hereditary origin. There are numerous other risk factors associated with the development of breast cancer. They may be classified as modifiable and non-modifiable risk factors. Modifiable risk factors are those that you can change by adopting a healthier lifestyle. Of course, you have no control over the non-modifiable risk factors, but awareness of these risks will definitely help in the early detection and diagnosis of breast cancer. We have already seen that early diagnosis has the multiple benefits of lower cost of treatment, lesser morbidity, and a higher chance of survival.

Non-Modifiable Risk Factors:

1. Gender: Women are more prone to developing breast cancer. Breast cancer can occur in men as well, but the incidence is not as high as seen in women.
2. Age: Breast cancer is seen more commonly in older women. The risk of developing breast cancer increases with age. Most breast cancers are seen in women aged 55 and older.
3. Gene Mutations: Breast cancer can be inherited through genetic mutations. These gene changes are thought to be directly passed on from a parent. It must be remembered that only five to ten percent of breast cancers are thought to have a genetic origin. The most common of these mutations occur in the *BRCA1* or the *BRCA2* genes. Normally these are genes that play a role in protein synthesis to repair damaged DNA. When the mutation occurs in these genes, it leads to abnormal cell growth and cancer.

Other genes involved are *PTEN*, *TP53*, *CDH1*, *STK11*, *CHEK2*, *BRIP1*, *ATM*, and *PALB2*. I will explain more about these later in the chapter.

4. Family History: Most women who develop breast cancer do not have a family history of the same. However, women who have close blood relatives with breast cancer do have a higher chance of developing breast cancer. If your first-degree relative, that is, mother, sister, or daughter, has breast cancer, then your risk of developing breast cancer doubles. If two first-degree relatives have breast cancer, then the risk increases three-fold. Women who have a close male member of the family with breast cancer, such as the father or brother, are also at a higher risk of developing breast cancer themselves.

5. Personal History: A woman who has had cancer in one breast is at a higher risk of developing new cancer in the other breast or in another part of the same breast. This risk is more pronounced in younger women who have been diagnosed with breast cancer.

6. Race and Ethnicity: Overall, white women are at a slightly higher risk of developing breast cancer than African-American women. But in women below the age of 40, the risk is higher in African-American women. Also, mortality from breast cancer is higher in African-American women. Studies show that Asian, Hispanic, and Native American women have a lower risk of developing breast cancer and a lower mortality rate as well.

7. Height: It has been found that taller women seem to be at a higher risk of developing breast cancer. The reason for this is still not clear, but hormonal and genetic factors and nutrition in early life are thought to play a role.

8. Dense Breasts: The breast is composed of fatty tissue, fibrous tissue, and glandular tissue. Breasts appear dense on the mammogram when they have more fibrous and glandular tissue and less fatty tissue.

Women who are seen to have dense breasts on mammography are at a higher risk for developing breast cancer than women whose breasts show normal density on the mammogram. The presence of dense breast tissue can also make it difficult to detect cancer at times. Breast density increases with age and in some other conditions, such as menopause and pregnancy.

9. Benign Breast Conditions: Certain types of non-cancerous breast diseases increase the risk of developing cancer. These benign conditions are classified into groups, depending on the risk they pose.

(a) Non-proliferative lesions—These include mild hyperplasia, fibrosis, simple cysts in the breast, adenosis, fat necrosis, and lipoma. These conditions have a very low risk of developing into cancer. Infection in the breast tissue is called mastitis, and this condition does not increase the risk of breast cancer.

(b) Proliferative lesions without atypia—There may be excessive growth of cells in the ducts and lobules of the breasts, but there are no abnormalities in the cells. These include conditions such as fibroadenoma, sclerosing adenosis, and ductal hyperplasia. These conditions increase the risk of breast cancer only slightly.

(c) Proliferative lesions with atypia—Here, the cells in the ducts or lobules of the breast grow excessively, and they look abnormal. This includes conditions such as atypical ductal hyperplasia and atypical lobular hyperplasia. Women who have these types of lesions have a four to five times higher chance of developing breast cancer. When in addition to having these atypical lesions, there is also a family history of breast cancer, the risk of developing breast cancer is even higher.

(d) Lobular carcinoma in situ (LCIS)—In this condition, cancer-like cells grow within the lobules of the milk-producing glands of the breast.

LCIS is not considered an invasive type of cancer as it does not spread beyond the lobule even if left untreated. However, women having LCIS are known to have a seven to twelve times higher risk of developing breast cancer in either breast.

10. Early Menarche: Women who started their menstrual cycles early, that is, before age 12, are known to have a slightly higher risk of developing breast cancer. The increased risk is attributed to having had more menstrual cycles and longer lifetime exposure to the estrogen and progesterone hormones.

11. Late Menopause: Here too the same principles of longer lifetime exposure to estrogen and progesterone and more menstrual cycles play a role in increasing the risk of developing breast cancer.

12. Radiation Exposure: Women who have been treated with radiation therapy to the chest in their childhood or adolescence for other cancers, such as Hodgkin or Non-Hodgkin lymphoma, have a higher risk of developing breast cancer. Radiation exposure to the chest in older women does not increase their chance of developing breast cancer.

13. Cancer of Ovary, Uterus, or Colon: Women who have had these cancers or who have a family history of a close relative with these cancers are at a higher risk of developing breast cancer.

Modifiable Risk Factors

1. Obesity: Being overweight after menopause increases the risk of developing breast cancer. In fact, women who gain excessive weight in their adulthood are at a higher risk of developing breast cancer.

2. Physical inactivity: Studies show that regular physical activity reduces breast cancer risk. This is especially true for menopausal women. Physical activity at least twice or thrice

a week is said to be beneficial in reducing the risk of breast cancer.

3. Alcohol intake: Drinking alcohol has been clearly linked to an increased risk of breast cancer. The risk increases with the amount of alcohol consumed.

4. Not having children: Women who do not have children (nulliparous) or those who have their first child after the age of 30 are at a higher risk of developing breast cancer. Experiencing many pregnancies and becoming pregnant at a young age has been shown to reduce breast cancer risk.

5. Not breastfeeding: Studies have suggested that breastfeeding may slightly lower breast cancer risk in women.

6. Hormonal birth control pills: Birth control pills are said to increase breast cancer risk. Women who use oral contraceptive pills (OCP) are at a higher risk of developing breast cancer than women who do not use OCPs. Other preparations such as long-acting depot progesterone injections and intrauterine devices that use hormones have also been suggested as increasing the risk of breast cancer, although there are no adequate studies to prove it.

7. Hormone therapy: Menopausal hormone therapy with estrogen and progesterone is used to relieve symptoms of menopause and prevent osteoporosis of the bones. The other term used is hormone replacement therapy (HRT). HRT is of two types: (a) Combined hormone therapy—estrogen and progesterone—is prescribed for women who still have a uterus. (b) Estrogen replacement therapy for women who have undergone a hysterectomy. Combined hormone therapy after menopause is said to increase the risk of breast cancer development. The risk associated with estrogen therapy is not very clear. Researchers say there may be a small risk of breast cancer in women who have been prescribed estrogen therapy.

Family History of Breast Cancer

The role of family history and genetics in breast cancer is not very well understood by many women. Some women believe that if there is no family history of breast cancer, they are sure not to get it. I would like to explain in detail the role of family history in breast cancer. As mentioned previously, there is a two-fold increase in the chances of developing breast cancer if a first-degree relative, such as the mother, sister, or daughter, has been diagnosed with breast cancer. This becomes more significant if the relative was diagnosed in the premenopausal period or if the cancer was bilateral. The risk is said to increase by 13.6 times if two first-degree relatives are affected.

In general, genetic factors are said to be responsible for only five percent to ten percent of breast cancers. However, in women aged below 30 years, they can account for up to 30 percent.

In families who have multiple affected members, especially when they are diagnosed with bilateral and early-onset cancer, the first-degree relatives are said to have a 50 percent absolute risk of developing breast cancer. The mode of inheritance is said to be autosomal dominant.

BRCA1 and BRCA2: Mutation in these genes is one of the common causes of inherited breast cancer. If you have inherited a mutated copy of one of these genes from a parent, you have a higher risk of developing breast cancer. A woman with a *BRCA1* or *BRCA2* gene mutation has a 7 in 10 chance of developing breast cancer by the age of 80. This risk increases if more than one family member is affected.

Women with either of these mutations are likely to be diagnosed with breast cancer at a younger age, and they are more likely to have involvement of both breasts.

Again, women with either of these mutations are also at a higher risk of developing ovarian cancer. The same applies to men as well. Men who inherit one of these gene changes are at a higher risk for breast cancer as well as some other cancers.

A few other gene mutations can also lead to inherited breast cancers. These mutations are less common and the risk of breast cancer is not as high as that associated with the *BRCA* genes.

ATM: The *ATM* gene normally helps in the repair of damaged DNA. Inheriting one abnormal copy of this gene has been linked to a high risk of breast cancer.

PALB2: The *PALB2* gene synthesizes a protein that interacts with the protein synthesized by the *BRCA2* gene. Mutations in this gene are said to lead to a higher risk of breast cancer.

TP53: The *TP53* gene helps to stop the growth of cells with damaged DNA. Inherited mutations of this gene cause the Li-Fraumeni syndrome. People with this syndrome have an increased risk of developing breast cancer along with other cancers, such as leukemia, brain tumors, and sarcomas (cancers of bones or connective tissue). This mutation is a rare cause of breast cancer.

CHEK2: The *CHEK2* gene normally helps with DNA repair. A mutation in this gene is said to increase breast cancer risk.

PTEN: The *PTEN* gene normally helps regulate cell growth. Inherited mutations in this gene can cause Cowden syndrome, a rare disorder that puts people at a higher risk of developing both malignant and benign tumors in the breasts, as well as growths in the digestive tract, thyroid, uterus, and ovaries.

CDH1: Inherited mutations in this gene cause a rare type of stomach cancer called hereditary diffuse gastric cancer. Women with mutations in this gene also have an increased risk of invasive lobular breast cancer.

STK11: Defects in this gene can lead to Peutz-Jeghers syndrome. People affected with this disorder have pigmented spots on their lips and in their mouths, polyps (abnormal growths) in the urinary and digestive tracts, and a higher risk of many types of cancer, including breast cancer.

Genetic Counseling and Testing

Genetic testing mainly looks for inherited mutations in the *BRCA1* and *BRCA2* genes. It is done less commonly for the other gene mutations. *BRCA1* mutations are said to be located on chromosome 17 and *BRCA2* mutations occur on chromosome 13. Women with these mutations are at an increased risk of not only breast cancer but also ovarian cancer.

There is an approximately 20 percent risk of a *BRCA1* mutation in a woman who has triple-negative breast cancer. In case there is a family history of breast and ovarian cancer in different relatives of a breast cancer patient, then there is approximately 40 percent risk of a *BRCA* gene mutation. If a relative has both breast and ovarian cancer, the risk can be as high as 80 percent. The *BRCA2* gene is located on chromosome 13[24] and accounts for 30 percent of familial breast cancers; in contrast to *BRCA1*, *BRCA2* is associated with increased breast cancer risk in men. Women with a mutation in *BRCA2* also have a 20 percent to 30 percent lifetime risk for ovarian cancer.

Genetic testing and counseling can help in the following situations:
- Diagnosis of breast cancer at a young age.
- Triple-negative breast cancer.
- Diagnosed with a second breast cancer.
- Family history of breast, ovarian, pancreatic, or prostate cancers.
- Family history of *BRCA* or other gene mutations.

[24]https://www.sciencedirect.com/topics/medicine-and-dentistry/chromosome-13

Gene testing can be done on a saliva sample, blood, or cancer tissue or block. Once the results are in, your doctor can best guide you on how to proceed. Some women with strong family history and *BRCA* mutations have opted to undergo a prophylactic bilateral mastectomy to reduce their chances of developing breast cancer. However, these decisions are usually made after adequate counseling. Women with gene mutations need to be monitored closely with adequate screening for cancer.

SURVIVOR NOTES

Name: Deepa Gupta
Age: 39
Location: Faizabad

Destiny often scripts some cryptic chapters for us, and we as humans end up getting a new definition altogether. My name is Deepa Gupta, and these days, I have got a new tagline behind my name: a breast cancer survivor. That is my new identity, and I do not lose any opportunity to tell people my story. I hope to bring a ray of hope to every person who has fallen prey to this dreadful cancer.

I was born on September 29, 1982, and am 39 years old. I live in Faizabad district in Uttar Pradesh and work as an assistant teacher in the Belser block in the neighboring Gonda district.

I have an elder sister who was diagnosed with breast cancer a few years ago, and I have watched her brave journey as she fought the disease and successfully triumphed over it. Perhaps this was the reason I was very aware of cancer and how it may present itself. The very word cancer definitely strikes a chord of fear in most people's hearts. But I am here to say that fearing a disease like cancer shall push one farther from its cure.

These days, medical science has crossed almost all barriers to finding new treatments to make breast cancer completely curable. An early diagnosis of certain cancers like breast cancer can lead to a completely cancer-free life. Mere awareness of the condition can help save many lives.

The first step in the battle against breast cancer is being aware. Identifying the symptoms at an early stage helps in combating the disease in a better way. I would say the battle is half won once the diagnosis is made.

In this modern era, we are exposed to so many harmful carcinogens in our food and products we use in our daily lives.

Carcinogens are cancer-producing compounds. It seems almost impossible to avoid these harmful chemicals. However, we can avoid everything that comes with a cautionary note, like tobacco products. Keeping ourselves healthy is in our hands. We are responsible for what we eat and what we practice in our daily lives. Avoiding harmful and toxic substances can help us in strengthening our immune systems.

As I had mentioned before, my sister won this battle against breast cancer. I was very aware of the possibility of a genetic predisposition to this disease. Basically, it means that breast cancer may run in families. One has to be more careful if your mother, sister, or mother's sisters were diagnosed with breast cancer at any time.

Of course, knowledge about cancer does not take away the scariness associated with the condition. When I first noticed bleeding from my right nipple, I was petrified. I could not feel any lump, but I was sure something was wrong. We immediately made an appointment to meet Dr. Anand Mishra at the King George's Medical University Hospital. I was asked to undergo some screening tests, such as mammography and ultrasound breast. The test results were clear. I was diagnosed to have early-stage cancer of the right breast. No matter how aware one is, you are bound to lose your composure once you are diagnosed with such a terrifying ailment. I, too, fell from the sky, holding a truck-load of whys and hows.

A lot of thoughts swirled through my mind. I started recollecting my sister's treatment. The very first thing that haunted me was the hair fall after chemotherapy. I didn't want to face that. No woman would ever want to meet such a horrifying sight. Long and luscious hair is ourfirst sign of beauty. No woman would agree to compromise on that. However, I couldn't sit and sink into those thoughts. I had to move on, and I soon came out of that phase.

I prepared myself mentally for the fight. Instead of glaring at the side effects, I sought courage from all those brave souls who gave a tough fight against the disease and won over it. After seeing my sister's successful journey, my family was confident that I could beat the disease. The tumor was very small and at an early stage; thus, I underwent surgery first. My main concerns were with the side effects of chemotherapy. However, following the surgery, the doctors said that chemotherapy wouldn't be necessary for me. That small ounce of consolation seemed like a blessing to me. I can confidently say the only reason for this good news was an early diagnosis. The doctors could catch hold of my breast cancer and nip it in the bud. And this was possible because of my awareness of the disease following my sister's diagnosis. I was also able to reach the right place for the right treatment. I cannot stress this enough. Experience and awareness were the main reasons behind my healing from cancer.

When I first noticed the bleeding, I did not hide it or delay in consulting the doctors for treatment. I immediately told my family, and without any further delay, I took the necessary steps to see the consultant for further tests and treatment. As a result, I am now leading a normal and healthy life. My message to all women is this: Be aware of your family history. If there is a history of breast cancer in the female members of your family, then your chances of getting the disease are also high. On the same note, you need not be scared of the facts. You should rather take all the precautionary measures and be vigilant toward any suspicious changes in your body. My only advice as a breast cancer survivor would be to shout out to every woman—Check your body regularly.

No change is small. A woman's body works on a multitude of hormones, and they can go wrong in any way possible.

Learn the proper way of performing breast self-examination. It is very important, and factually, one can identify small-sized lumps at an early stage itself.

Remember, early diagnosis and treatment of breast cancer will most definitely increase your chances of a cancer-free life.

Similarly, I would also request those women who have been diagnosed with breast cancer and are undergoing treatment to share their experiences with family and friends. We often keep our problems only within the close family and do not share them with the extended family. Being diagnosed with breast cancer is not a crime, and neither is it a shameful thing. Rather the other women in your family must be aware so that they can be careful and get themselves checked if necessary. On my part, I make it a point to talk about my journey with all my colleagues. I teach how to perform breast self-examination to those who wish to learn the right way to do it. I tell people that cancer is not scary. It is not the end, and there are lots of new and advanced treatments available.

My Block Education Officer has encouraged me to visit different schools in our area and speak to the female members of the staff. I encourage the women to maintain a healthy weight and exercise regularly.

I am forever grateful for the support and encouragement of my doctor and all the staff at King George's Medical University. My family stood by me consistently and never allowed me to lose hope. I am thankful to them. My husband was a pillar of strength and took care of all my appointments and the household chores as well during my surgery and recovery. My two young children, Soham and Kavya, who are just seven and five years of age, respectively, gave me a lot of positivity.

My doctors declared me cancer-free on June 25, 2018, and that day shall always remain etched in my memory. I consider it as my day of reincarnation. I have been given a new lease on life. I am a proud breast cancer survivor!

Women with a positive family history of breast cancer should undergo periodic screening.
Check your body regularly. No change is small.

Deepa Gupta had a family history of breast cancer. Because her sister had been diagnosed earlier and had undergone treatment for the same, she was vigilant.

In her own words, awareness and experience played a key role in her early diagnosis. Because of her awareness of the significance of family history and her knowledge about breast cancer, Deepa sought immediate treatment when she noticed her own symptoms. Her cancer was identified in stage 1 and she successfully completed her treatment. Deepa attributes her cancer-free status to early diagnosis and treatment. Another important point she makes is involving the other family members. If a woman is diagnosed with breast cancer, it is important that the other close female members of the family are aware of it.

Allowing others in the family to know about your diagnosis can make them aware of the condition. It helps them be vigilant toward their own health. In fact, they can be taught to perform breast self-examination and also encouraged to undergo a mammogram every two years. Having survived breast cancer, Deepa takes her responsibilities seriously. She is keen to tell of her experience to people and encourages women to take their health seriously. Spreading awareness about breast cancer is very much needed in our society. And when a cancer survivor speaks, the impact is so much more.

Till now, I have shared the stories of many women who have survived breast cancer. However, breast cancer can also affect men. Here is the story of a very brave male patient, a motor mechanic, who fought this cancer successfully. He died in late 2021 due to chronic kidney failure during the second wave of the pandemic, when we doctors were struggling with Covid, and non-Covid services were suboptimal.

Name: Mehtab Khan
Age: 50 years
Location: Lucknow

The year 2016 has brought some dramatic and drastic changes in my life. My name is Mehtab Khan, and it was the first time in my life that I had spent 15 days in a hospital.

Soon, due to *Bakri Eid*, I was sent back home to celebrate my religious festival. Once it was over, I paid a visit to Dr. Anand Mishra in the Medical College. I was advised for a biopsy for an ulcerated lesion/wound on the right chest near the nipple and I got it done from a very reputed pathological center. The reports took 15 days to come. The doctor asked me to get admitted on seeing the reports. However, Diwali was impending, so I was again sent back home. Once I got admitted, my treatment procedure was initiated. A chunk was cut out of my breast and was sent for analysis. The reports proved it to be cancerous. The first course of treatment started with chemotherapy. After every 21 days, I was administered chemotherapy drugs. I lost all my hair after two sessions of chemotherapy. My surgery was performed after six sessions of chemotherapy. After chemotherapy, I underwent surgery on the chest wall. Later, Dr. Mishra suggested radiation therapy, where I had to undergo 17 sessions.

I have never heard of a man suffering from breast cancer before, but during my treatment, I came across a few in the hospital. I will advise all men to be vigilant about any changes in their nipple or chest wall. Cancer is curable and it is evident from my story. Never lose hope and be a warrior, whatever comes in your life. In my whole course of treatment, all my problems were attended to well. I shall always remain indebted to all the doctors of the endocrine surgery department at KGMU, and all the other hospital staff for helping me out at every stage of treatment.

Men too can develop breast cancer.
Never lose hope and be a warrior, whatever comes in your life.

Unlike the various women who have narrated their stories with all their thoughts and emotions poured in, Mehtab's recording of his breast cancer story is sort of emotionless and to the point. However, his story serves to highlight the important fact that men too can be affected by breast cancer, and they too need to be vigilant.

How does breast cancer occur in men? Men have breast tissue too. Until puberty, the breast tissue is similar in girls and boys. At puberty, the female hormones cause breast ducts to grow and lobules to form in the girls. However, in boys, the amount of breast tissue remains the same as before. There may be few ducts and almost no lobules. These ducts are not functional in men, but at times breast cancer can originate from these ducts and the glands in the male breast. Cancer may present as pain in the breast or a breast lump or swelling. In men, too, breast cancer spreads through the lymphatic system with the axillary lymph nodes being the first to be affected. The risk factors for men to develop breast cancer are family history and inherited gene mutations. It has been found that 1 out of 5 men with breast cancer have a close male or female relative who has been diagnosed with breast cancer. The risk is higher with *BRCA2* mutations than that with *BRCA1* mutations. The other risk factors are radiation exposure, alcohol abuse, liver disease such as cirrhosis, obesity, and estrogen therapy given for prostate cancer. Apart from a lump, breast cancer in men can present with skin dimpling, nipple retraction, redness or scaling of the nipple or skin, or discharge from the nipple. In advanced stages, axillary swelling of the lymph nodes may be detected. Diagnosis is based on biopsy and imaging studies. Hormone receptor status is studied, and HER2 status is identified as well to decide if targeted therapy is required. When diagnosed early, male breast cancer patients have a very good five-year survival rate.

I would like to reiterate that being aware of the risk factors for developing breast cancer plays a huge role in early diagnosis and treatment.

Women who have a family history of breast cancer should ensure that they go for periodic screening. Not having a family history does not mean you will not develop breast cancer. Be aware of the modifiable risk factors such as obesity, alcohol abuse, etc., and ensure healthy lifestyle practices. Men too need to be vigilant. If you have the slightest doubt, please get it checked immediately. Early diagnosis of breast cancer improves survival rates enormously as is obvious from Deepa's story.

9

NEW NORMAL AFTER CURE

Facing the future with hope

The one thing uppermost in a cancer survivor's mind on completion of the treatment is the relief of completing the treatment. However, that is not the only emotion that they would be feeling. Most cancer survivors would have a mixed bag of emotions to deal with, and breast cancer survivors are no different. They would be grateful for the timely diagnosis and treatment they had received. They would be excited to move on with their lives, but they would still have anxiety about what the future holds in store for them.

Along with the joy and relief at the successful completion of treatment, fear and worry remain constant companions for every cancer survivor. What is the new normal going to be like? What can you expect?

A breast cancer survivor has been through a lot in the course of her treatment. She has literally been through a roller coaster of emotions as she underwent the treatment.

Most survivors look forward to returning to their old lives and picking up from where they left them.

Some women take this opportunity to reassess their life and lifestyle and figure out what is important now for them and what no longer holds any significance.

So, why exactly is this period called a 'new normal?' How different is it from the old lifestyle or life patterns that you had before your diagnosis? And does it have to be a 'new normal' for every cancer survivor? Come, let us explore some of these concerns and find out more about the life that a cancer survivor can look forward to.

The Australian actor and singer Alyssa-Jane Cook once said: *Breast cancer changes you, and the change can be beautiful!* The change from being a cancer patient to becoming a cancer survivor is different for each person. Some patients consider themselves to be cancer survivors right from the time their diagnosis was confirmed because they are proactively going forward with the therapy, and they choose to view the whole exercise from a positive viewpoint.

Many others consider themselves to be cancer survivors when their therapy is completed and when they are declared cancer-free by their doctors. The term 'survivor' by itself is a strong word. It indicates struggle, fight, winning, hope, and much more. It is a positive term.

However, there are some people who do not wish to be identified in any way after the completion of their treatment. It is their choice as they are probably dealing with a lot of negative feelings or guilt. Whatever the term or label of reference, it cannot be disputed that patients who have successfully completed their cancer therapy and have been declared cancer-free have indeed been through a lot. All through the period of treatment, patients feel like their life is on hold. And once the treatment is complete, they look forward to quickly getting back on their feet and carrying on with their lives as before.

The sad truth is that it is often not possible to do this. Cancer and its treatment exact quite a toll not only on the individual but also on the family. Cancer survivors experience changes in many aspects.

Their appearance is changed, their thought processes are different post-therapy, and their functional status may be changed as well.

Getting back to mainstream life may sometimes involve making changes to your life patterns or adopting new methods of coping.

It takes some time, but cancer survivors can slowly find a new way of living and coping—the new normal.

Transition to the New Normal

Life after cancer therapy is all about making adjustments and accepting yourself. Your body and your mind have been through a highly stressful experience, and you need time to recover from the stress and pain of the diagnosis, treatment, and procedures. Immediately after completing the cancer treatment, you can go through a confusing state of mind. You may even experience feelings of guilt that you are not back on your feet as expected. You may feel you are letting your family down.

Coping with the changes takes time, and each person is unique in that respect. This new normal may include changes in the food you eat, dealing with scars on your body, difficulty in doing certain activities that you could easily do before, financial constraints that were not there previously, and emotional changes from going through the cancer ordeal. Some cancer survivors are able to accept the 'new normal' easily and settle into the new pattern of life easily. However, it takes a long time for some others to get over the trauma of treatment and the memories of their previous normal life.

There is no particular timeframe for this transition. You do not have to adapt by a certain day or date. Some people may adapt easily. For some, it may take a long time before they get used to the new life. You may think you are a different person now, or others may think you are different.

The common thing faced by most cancer survivors is uncertainty—uncertainty about cancer coming back or moving forward in life in general. Another common emotion faced by survivors is loss of control of their life. What is important is that you give yourself enough time to assimilate your thoughts and the changes that have taken place. Take life one day at a time.

Cancer Can be a Life-Changing Experience

Almost all breast cancer survivors refer to their experience as a life-changing one. Some even find to their surprise that there are some positive aspects. Cancer survivors find an inner strength that they did not know they possessed. It is this inner strength that helped them fight the disease successfully. Cancer may make you question your priorities in life. What you thought was important may no longer seem as important now. As a cancer survivor, you will find yourself giving more importance to friendships and family relationships. Some people decide to travel and see more of the world or start a new enterprise. Most cancer survivors look forward to making positive lifestyle changes, such as reducing stress in their lives or exercising regularly. Often, survivors want to give back to society or other cancer patients, and they look for ways in which they can do so. However, remember there is no hurry. Focus on your recovery, both physical and emotional. Once you are well enough, you can go forward to help others. There is plenty of time.

Role of the Healthcare Team

From the time of the diagnosis of breast cancer, all the decisions regarding your health would have been made by others. When the treatment is complete, patients can feel a sense of abandonment as now they suddenly feel they are left without support. Another fear is that of recurrence. Any suggestive symptoms that you experience will give rise to the fear of cancer re-occurring. Talk to your doctor about your fears. Talking out about your fears will help to calm your fears. Fear of recurrence is normal, and it will slowly decrease with time. One of the ways to cope with this fear is to take control of your health. You can do this by becoming better informed about cancer recurrence. I have some suggestions that you can follow:

(a) Talk to your doctor: Confess your fears about cancer coming back to your doctor. Your doctor will tell you that the chance of recurrence is not the same for every breast cancer patient. You can learn about your type of cancer and the risk of recurrence specific to you.

(b) It is okay to be anxious: All cancer survivors start to worry when they experience any new ache or pain. Various aches and pains are normal after surgery and radiation therapy. However, make it a point to discuss with your doctor, who can allay your fears. Do not keep your fears to yourself as that is not good for your mental health.

(c) Keep a note of your concerns: Many patients find it helpful to record their symptoms as they appear. This will help you in conveying your concerns to the doctor during your next follow-up visit, and at the same time, it will also help to reduce your anxiety.

(d) Talk to a professional counselor: Many cancer survivors benefit from talking about their fears to a professional counselor. If the thought of cancer recurrence is occupying your mind enough to disturb your daily life, then professional counseling will help you.

(e) Maintain a proper follow-up schedule: Along with your oncologist, draw up a follow-up schedule. In the first few years, it might be six-monthly visits. The duration will be longer as time progresses. Having a regular schedule will help greatly in allaying fears of breast cancer recurrence. A good follow-up care plan not only addresses the cancer treatment and follow-up schedule but also includes suggestions to meet the emotional, social, or financial needs of the patient.

The follow-up care schedule depends upon the type of cancer, the treatment given, and the patient's overall health.

(f) Keep the connections: Never stop meeting, talking, and laughing with your friends, family, relatives, and people with whom you are comfortable.

(g) Keep active: Participate in activities that stimulate you and provide pleasure.
(h) Give back: Participate in voluntary social work.
(i) Join the team: Join the local breast cancer support group. If there is no support group in your city, take the step to create one.

Look After Yourself

It is important that you focus your energy on keeping your mind and body healthy and well. Whether cancer comes back or not is not in your hands. However, there are many steps that you can take to keep your mind free from worry and to rebuild your physical resilience.

(a) Learn to relax: Relaxation techniques such as meditation and yoga can help greatly reduce stress in your life. Experiment with various methods and find the best method to reduce your worry and stress.
(b) Share your feelings: Do not keep your emotions bottled up. Share your thoughts and fears with close friends and relatives. Opening up to others helps relieve stress within you.
You will be surprised by how many of your friends are open to listening and providing emotional support. The other option is to join various support groups. Here you will find others who are going through the same thing as you.
(c) Get out of your home: You were probably confined to your home through the long months of cancer therapy. Make a conscious effort to get back into society. Go out and attend functions and learn to enjoy the company of friends and relatives again.
This may not be the solution for everyone. You should not force yourself if you feel you are not ready, but try to make a small start.

(d) Look for spiritual help: Many cancer survivors talk about how spirituality helped them cope with the disease. Many of them talk about renewing their faith or religion. This can be your source of strength too.

(e) Get started on a healthy diet: During the various treatment rounds, you probably would not have been able to eat well as your appetite would have been low. Now is the time to build up your physical stamina and strength by going on a healthy diet. It is best to take the help of a dietitian or nutritionist who can guide you properly about the foods you should eat.

(f) Begin exercising: Exercise is known to be a mood elevator. Exercising enhances your sense of well-being. For cancer survivors, even moderate exercise can help reduce anxiety and depression. It can build up your self-esteem and boost your immunity as well. Studies have reported that low- to moderate-intensity home-based physical exercise helps relieve cancer fatigue significantly.

(g) Journaling: Maintaining a journal helps you put your thoughts down on paper. This has benefits beyond being able to discuss your worries with your doctor. When you write down your anxieties and thoughts or your fears about the future, you will find that they no longer hold the same grip over you. Journaling helps you get rid of your fears and anxieties.

(h) Take part in voluntary work: Being involved in social causes has the double benefit of turning your attention away from yourself and helping others. Cancer survivors feel like they have lost control of their lives, and others would have been helping them in many different ways. After your treatment, when you start helping others, it gives you a sense of worth. It can be a big boost to your identity and independence.

(i) Get involved in your follow-up: Cancer survivors say that getting actively involved in their follow-up care goes a long way in building their confidence. They feel that they are finally in control of their lives. Be involved actively in making plans, lifestyle changes, and important decisions about the future.

Follow-Up Plan After Cancer Therapy

The importance of having a regular follow-up schedule cannot be stressed enough. Follow-up examinations and testing can pick up cancer recurrence as soon as it happens.

Regular follow-up allows you to not live in fear of cancer recurring.

(a) Learn about the signs and symptoms of local and regional breast cancer recurrence. Practice breast self-examination monthly in between doctor visits.

(b) It is recommended that you go for a detailed cancer-related history and physical examination every three to six months for the first three years after your therapy. Thereafter, your doctor might recommend that you come in for a check-up every 6 to 12 months. The frequency of the follow-up visits depends on the type and stage of cancer that you had.

(c) Your doctor might recommend that you undergo annual mammography of the other breast if you had undergone a mastectomy and both breasts if you had undergone breast conservation surgery.

(d) Your doctor might ask you to undergo some other lab tests as well as an ultrasound scan of the breast as and when required.

(e) If you are on hormonal therapy, it is important to continue the same. Ask your doctor about how to manage the symptoms of hormonal therapy.

(f) It is important for the other family members to be aware of family history and take precautionary measures such as regular self-breast examination, annual clinical examination, and annual mammography.

How Can You Improve Your Diet?

It is important that once the cancer therapy is complete, you eat well. A proper diet can help regain your lost strength. It can help rebuild your muscles and tissues and help you feel better too. A nutritionist is the best person to help you plan a nutritious and balanced diet sheet. They will help you address any special dietary needs that you might have. Make sure that your diet plan includes food that you can actually eat. Try to include a variety of food from all the food groups. Make sure to include fruits, vegetables, whole grains, and protein in your diet in the right quantities. High-fiber foods like whole-grain bread are a good choice. It is better to avoid the consumption of red meat and alcohol. Studies have shown that including omega-3 fatty acid supplements in the diet resulted in better health in cancer survivors. Maintaining a healthy weight is also vital. A healthy and balanced diet contributes to overall wellness.

For Mastectomy Patients: Acquire a properly matched and sized breast prosthesis and wear it when you go out in public. It will improve your self-esteem.

Myth-Busters

There are a lot of myths associated with recovery from cancer as well. I want to address a few of them here.

(a) I should be normal: It does not work that way. A cancer patient cannot get back to normal the day the treatment stops. It is a process that you go through emotionally and physically.

(b) I should be positive: No one can be positive all the time, least of all someone who has been through the turmoil of breast cancer diagnosis and treatment. This is an unrealistic expectation. Do not let yourself be pushed into this thought. Take your time to recover.

There may be days when you are emotionally low and some days when you are in a more positive frame of mind.

(c) I should feel healthy: Intense therapy for cancer such as chemo and radiation therapy can leave a lot of side effects that are felt long after the completion of treatment. The body and mind take a long time to recover from the ordeal. The effects of treatment can affect your everyday life to a great extent.

(d) I do not need any more support: Cancer survivors require as much support on completion of treatment as they did when they were undergoing the treatment.

(e) I should be thankful: This is a reasonable expectation by everyone around you. Surviving breast cancer is indeed a big deal, but we should remember that cancer survivors often struggle with feelings of anger and resentment.

(f) I should celebrate: Some cancer survivors look upon each milestone in their treatment as an achievement worthy of celebration. But some others have feelings of guilt and confusion in their minds. It is not wrong to feel so; take your own time to get into the thankful or celebratory phase.

(g) I should go back to who I was: This is possibly the biggest myth that can stress out a cancer survivor completely. As we have seen, a survivor goes through so much trauma that it is almost impossible to become the same person. The focus should be on becoming a 'New You.' It is important to take life one day at a time. Recognize that there may be good days when you feel you can cope, and there may be bad days when you feel you cannot. In time, there will be more of the good days to look forward to.

SURVIVOR NOTES

Name: Kalpana Agarwal
Age: Undisclosed
Location: Pilibhit

Kalpana was beginning to feel more exhausted than usual. She attributed it to her increasing obligations at work without giving it much thought. But what happened after? Kalpana Agarwal, a mother of two, explains: Initially, I just assumed I was unwell. However, as I continued to feel tired, I began to get a little worried, and taking the matter a bit seriously, I scheduled an appointment with my doctor. And here I was, sitting in a stupor in a corridor of the Sanjay Gandhi Post Graduate Institute of Medical Sciences (PGI) in Lucknow, on what was perhaps the saddest day of my life. I had just been told that I had cancer. My initial reaction was one of absolute terror. I was convinced I was going to die. And then I started feeling sorry for myself. Indulging in self-pity, I wondered, "Why me?" What did I do to deserve this? I was also experiencing that all-too-familiar feeling of denial, as I sincerely prayed the report was not mine and that it was sent to me by mistake.

At that time, I was bewildered about how my life would be from now on. I have two sons, and the younger one was in his second year of college. My husband, too, had recently undergone cardiac bypass surgery. Everything seemed dark before me and the future seemed bleak. How would my family cope with this? My family was completely dependent on me, and I knew my life was invaluable to my children and my husband. My heart ached for my eldest son, who is very emotionally attached to me. It was my husband who gave me strength at this time. He consoled me, and I pulled myself together and composed myself. I knew I had to be strong to face this.

I was diagnosed with breast cancer following a biopsy at PGI. I had read somewhere that Cancer, in all of its manifestations, was one of the most serious worldwide health problems, in both this century and the previous one.

And the commonest cancer in women is breast cancer, especially in India. I recalled that from 2012, I had been feeling a bit light-headed and suffocated toward the end of the day, and this feeling persisted even after I came home from work. I also noticed that my breast size had gradually increased, and I wondered if I was gaining weight and would become obese. But at that time, I had absolutely no clue that it was the beginning of cancer growth in my breast. After a few days, I felt a small lump in my breast; there was no pain, but my uneasiness increased. I got frightened and told my husband about it. Ever since I felt the lump, I could not even sleep at night and felt very restless too. The word 'Cancer' brings fear to all those who hear it, and I tried to avoid thinking about it. However, the fear was lurking in some corner of my mind. I used to tell my husband that I had nowhere to go and no one else.

My husband took me to a private hospital in Bareilly in 2013. I underwent an ultrasound of the breast, but the sonography report did not mention a clear diagnosis. Following this, we started treatment from one of the most reputed homeopathic doctors in our country, although my fears remained. The doctor assured us that it was possible to completely cure my cancer through homeopathic treatment, and added that I should not panic at all.

My husband and I believed his words and started the treatment. The treatment lasted for about a year and a half, and then I noticed about two to three inflammatory areas on the breast externally. This made me panic and I immediately told my husband. We went to see a doctor in the local district hospital, and my husband narrated my symptoms and showed him the previous reports. He immediately advised us to go to PGI, and hence we arrived at Lucknow. As I mentioned before, the diagnosis of breast cancer was confirmed at PGI Lucknow.

Eventually, all my relatives and friends came to know about it as I had a lot of relatives staying in Lucknow. One of my cousins asked me to take Dr. Anand Mishra's opinion. Two days later, I reached King George's Medical University (KGMU) to meet Dr. Anand.

We showed him all my medical reports from PGI. He examined me thoroughly and went through all the test reports as well. He said that he was not happy with the biopsy done earlier and wanted it to be repeated. The second biopsy result showed that I now had Stage 3 grade 4 cancer. When I heard this, it felt like the ground gave way beneath my feet. I failed to see any ray of hope for my survival. However, the doctor consoled me and explained that breast cancer was very common in women. He assured me that it was treatable and asked me to be confident and not worry about it. He motivated me to be courageous and face the battle. I then composed and strengthened myself mentally for the sake of my home and children; I decided in my mind that I would overcome this disease by all means. I realized that the crucial word to remember while dealing with cancer is 'CAN'...that I can do it and conquer it. We must keep in mind that our mindset is the most significant factor in this fight against cancer.

On August 19, 2014, my treatment began at KGMU. On the same day as my biopsy, I also had a catheter inserted. This would help in infusing all the chemotherapy drugs without having to find a vein each time. This catheter cost around rupees 25,000, but more than the cost, the pain associated with the procedure was significant. I started my pre-chemo medications on August 20, 2014, and the first chemotherapy session was on August 21, 2014. After the chemo, I came home and lay silently on the bed with my eyes closed that day and started taking the name of the Lord. I said, "Oh God, now you are the only one who cares for me and can help me." I was unable to express in words the pain I was feeling from head to toe. On the fourth day, my brother sent me by car to Pilibhit, where I live. I still remember that journey as it was also very painful, but I never let my pain dominate my mind. I made the decision to go from "victim" to "victorious" mode.

With the correct mindset, I was sure I could defeat the 'beast.' I promised it that I was going to live—happily and meaningfully.

I was quite aware that I would be facing the many side-effects of chemotherapy shortly.

Fatigue is one of the predominant and common side effects following chemotherapy. It is a deep-seated tiredness where you feel like you will never be able to do anything again. The doctor had warned me about the other more tangible side-effects of chemo, such as cessation of menstruation and hair loss. Sure enough, my periods stopped after my first chemotherapy session, and I developed multiple ulcers in my mouth. This too was a result of the chemo drugs. The taste sensations were gone; I could just about taste anything sweet. After the chemo, there was severe constipation, which was followed by severe diarrhea. The chemo cycles were scheduled for every 21 days, and before each cycle, I had to do a blood test. This was to check my platelet count. The platelet count was normal, and when I reached the hospital for the second round of chemo, we heard some encouraging progress: The size of the lump in my breast had decreased from 4 4 cm to 3.5 cm. My second chemotherapy session was on September 8, 2014.

I was somehow carrying within me the ability to bear the pain after every chemo, but I was completely broken on the day my hair loss began. When my hair started to fall out, I started crying bitterly because I had not even dreamed that there would come a time when I would not have hair on my head. This situation shook my heart to the core. Despite these difficult events, I did not let my self-confidence break in any way because I knew that if my morale were broken, I would never be able to recover from cancer. I kept praying to the Almighty and constantly reminded myself that I had to live for my family.

For me, completing each chemo session was like winning a big battle! The third chemotherapy session was on September 29, 2014, and the size of the lump was now 2.5 cm. Following the chemo, I experienced the same painful cycle, and I had to repeat the same seven-day medication routine.

However, this time the drugs affected my teeth as well: the upper crust of the enamel started falling from my teeth. I lost all sense of taste and could hardly taste anything properly. I used to take a spoonful of porridge in my mouth and add a little milk or some almonds to make it a little tasty.

I forced myself to eat because I knew I had to keep my strength up. I gave up looking at the mirror because I used to find my face very strange without hair and it was distressing to me. In the meantime, I started developing shivers, which were quite bad, and this new symptom was quite awful. We went to see Dr. Mishra, who examined me and said that the catheter had become infected. He immediately had it removed.

Now, this meant that a new catheter had to be inserted each time I went for chemotherapy. This procedure was also very difficult for me because my veins were not prominent, and I had to suffer a lot. I underwent the fourth chemo on October 28, 2014. By this time, I had lost all appetite and was not eating much. Physically, I was very weak. Also, the various medicines that were being absorbed by my body as part of pre-chemo and the chemo drugs were together causing a lot of new symptoms. The chemo drugs were usually prescribed based on the body weight. I completed the fifth and sixth chemo cycles on November 21, 2014, and December 11, 2014, respectively. I realized that after every chemo cycle, my pain was increasing, such as pain in the stomach and severe pain in the legs. I had to wait for a while even to stand up. Only the almighty knows how difficult it was for me as I used to take my time and pause before returning home. On my way back home after chemo, my legs used to tremble for a long time, and by the time I could walk, my throat used to be dry. It was so dry that no matter how much water I drank, it remained the same. For this reason, I used to keep cardamom and bubblegum in my mouth all the time. I used to sit awake all night and just pray to the Lord to give me life for the sake of my children. The pain was ever-present, but I was ready to face all these challenges just in the hope of staying alive. Next, I was scheduled to undergo an operation. My surgery also took place in the bitter winter.

I had to travel by train from Lucknow to Pilibhit The train used to leave at 12.00 midnight, and during the winter season, it was never on time. We usually had to wait at the station for more than an hour. There were no vehicles available at night, and we usually had to call someone, either a relative or a friend, to drive our car.

They would pick us up from the station, drop us at our doorstep, and then return to their own homes. They never complained or considered it a chore but rather did it out of empathy and love. Later I underwent radiotherapy. The radiotherapy sessions lasted for 23 days, and after that, we returned to Pilibhit after completing my check-up. Next, I was planned for targeted therapy, three weekly cycles. It started in April 2015. And the doctors advised the same precautions: avoid exposure to sun and dust, drink more water. Some hair had regrown in the intervening period, but I still did not dare to see my face in the mirror. I had a fear of losing them again. The scarf remained firmly tied around my head.

I finished the therapy in July 2015. Based on the final reports, I was further advised to have hormone tablets for five years. Although these medicines had many side effects and caused me many physical problems, I did not lose my morale. I developed my mental resilience and controlled my mind. I made myself think this way: When I have managed to overcome such a deadly disease, why should I worry about these side effects? My body has just been subjected to a massive attack and healing is crucial. It is true that I am not going to get back on my feet immediately, but get back, I will. Today, I feel like a victor who defeated death in the battle between life and death and won the gold medal of life!

Alternative therapies do more harm than good, as in my case.
Cancer is 'CAN'...that I can do it and conquer it.

The most important learning from Kalpana's success story is about the consequence of not believing the diagnosis and beginning the treatment. In fact, she moved to Homeopathy and delayed her treatment for more than a year.

This led to progression in the cancer stage. If she had commenced the treatment early, she probably would not have undergone so much pain. I am happy that she survived the fight. Kalpana is aware that the road back to recovery is going to be steep. She talks about the various side effects of medicines that she has to continue taking for five more years. But she does not sound disheartened. That is the important part—to recognize that your journey back will be different, and the routine you get back to will be different as well. There is no hurry to get back on your feet; rather, take the time to allow both your mind and body to recover.

Survivorship after breast cancer is a marathon, not a sprint. That includes applying the adaptive methods learned while on chemotherapy or recuperating from surgery to deal with symptoms that persist after treatment has ended. It is necessary to continue to schedule periods of rest and be aware of the specific activities that make one most weary. If you feel that your symptoms of mental fog persist, you can use methods such as writing things down, leaving reminders to yourself, and requesting individuals to repeat information. Everyone, not just you, is eager for the completion of the treatment. Although all your friends and family have been extremely supportive, they may want you to bounce back right away when you stop treatment. Unfortunately, this takes time, and it is a slow process where you learn what is best for you. Take your time. There is no time limit for your recovery.

Christina Steinorth-Powell, the noted psychotherapist and author says, *"Have your own experience and trust your intuition. A million people will tell you what you should and shouldn't be doing, but you know yourself and your body best—do what you think is right."*

Here I am repeating some tips that can help you cope in this period after you have completed your cancer therapy:
- Take it one day at a time.
- Develop small wellness goals.
- Share your thoughts with family and friends.
- Be involved in your follow-up.

- Do things at your own pace.
- Write down your thoughts in a journal.
- Do not give in to pressure from others or to their unrealistic expectations.
- Ask for help: you do not have to do it all alone.
- Read about or meet others who have been on this journey.
- Eat a balanced diet.
- Make sure you get to exercise every day.
- Practice meditation or yoga.
- Tell yourself what you are going through is 'normal'—the 'new normal.'

There is life ahead after surviving cancer. Maybe it is going to be a bit different from what you have been used to, but it will be a beautiful one, nevertheless.

10

A MESSAGE FROM THE SURVIVORS

Looking forward with hope

You have been reading the different stories of women who have successfully battled breast cancer and have come out victorious. Each of their journeys was different.

Their family circumstances were different. They were of different ages. The stage at which breast cancer was diagnosed was different as well.

However, the one common shining thread you see running through each of these stories is the courage and determination with which these warriors faced their disease. So, it is very important not to give up or give in to despair.

The former US President Theodore Roosevelt is known to have said,

"Believe you can, and you're halfway there."

It is true indeed! Believing you will prevail against cancer is half the battle won. That is not to say it is going to be an easy fight.

But going in with hope and courage will definitely help you in your journey. In fact, many doctors now prefer not to use the terms 'fight' or 'battle.' After all, cancer, including breast cancer, is a disease that does not always respond to therapy the way we think it should. There is always a factor of uncertainty with cancer. The patient is not entirely in control of what happens to her. But stepping into the treatment regimen with a positive mindset definitely helps.

Let us not worry about the semantics, I say. It is enough for a breast cancer patient to try to survive and thrive through her therapy. And for this, I want to leave you with thoughts shared by my cancer survivors based on their experiences. These confessions of cancer survivors will help you or your dear ones cope when they face the same situation.

1. "It is very important to keep your mind occupied with positive thoughts and activities."
2. "You never know how strong you are until being strong is the only choice you have."
3. "It is okay to be afraid, but remember that you are not alone in this fight. Positivity, strength, courage, indomitable spirit, and confidence are the key ingredients in this fight."
4. "Never give up. Miracles can and do happen. Believe that you will be cured and you will come out a winner."
5. "Realize that feeling feminine or sexy need not depend on the size of your breasts or on whether your breasts remain or have been removed. Your femininity goes much deeper."
6. "Do not worry too much or overthink the situation. Learn to stay calm. Tell yourself that what is happening is for the good. Learn to live in the moment."
7. "Do not believe everything you read on Google. There is a lot of misinformation that can be harmful."

8. "You will find inner strength that you never knew you had. This will help you become a conqueror."

9. "Every human has an inner strength that they need to use to fight this."

10. "Tell yourself this: I will do anything and everything to stay alive, and I will make sure that this has the least impact on my life."

11. "Cancer no longer rules or dictates my life. I have conquered it, and I will continue to fight the myths associated with it."

12. "After mastectomy, I do not feel any less of a woman. It has not diminished my femininity."

13. "When I first came to know that I had breast cancer, I was scared and broken. The only thought I had was 'I want to be cured of cancer and I do not really care what my body will look like.' Now, when I have been cured, I do not mind my scars or my appearance. I feel stronger and more powerful and more confident."

14. "Well, I have conquered it; I do not know how I did it. What can I say? I am truly grateful. But of course, it is more than that. I feel like a newborn woman now."

15. "This can happen to anyone. But if you are practicing self-examination or if you go to your doctor for a clinical examination as soon as you experience any breast symptoms, cancer can be diagnosed early. That would be incredible."

16. "I am a fairly educated active woman. But I knew very little about breast care or monthly breast self-examination until I was diagnosed with breast cancer. I want to tell other women that practicing breast self-examination can help in the early identification of the problem."

17. "Few things that I learned from my illness: Keep your health first and take care of yourself. Do not try to make everybody happy. I also learned that however much you think you can control events in life, you really cannot."

18. "I was perfectly happy and healthy and did not have any family history of breast cancer. But I had breast cancer. So, some things just happen. You just have to face the facts and fight it."

19. "Cancer diagnosis made me feel alone and scared. But my support group is a network of amazing and good people, and they helped me cope and win over it."

20. "I was worried about my children and family. My doctor assured me saying, 'You will be there to see them grow.' Early detection is the key to curing breast cancer. That is why women need to undergo yearly mammograms, and they should have awareness as well."

21. "Family support is important and I am lucky that I had it. It was tough to see women who did not have that support. Always face challenges with a brave face."

22. "Cancer was like a big wave, and it passed. But it turned out to be a blessing. It gave me a new perspective, incredible clarity, and a lot of peace."

23. "Everyone has their own story. Everyone has been through ups and downs. I think what stands out for me the most is just the love, care, and support of my family and friends."

24. "Accept what is, let go of what was, and have faith in what will be. Surround yourself with only people who are going to lift you higher. Cancer is a word, not a sentence."

I believe that these words of breast cancer survivors can bring hope, courage, strength, belief, and confidence to breast cancer patients. Let their words and experiences transform your thoughts and beliefs into positive ones. Let me leave you with the words of the inspirational writer Jonathan Lockwood Huie:

"Miracles are the natural way of the universe. Our only job is to move our doubting minds out of the way."

CONCLUSION

A lot has been written on the various aspects of breast cancer, but there are many points that merit more attention and directed action. Significant progress has been made in increasing awareness about breast cancer amongst women, but the same does not hold true for male breast cancer.

The male population needs to be sensitized about this disease as they are directly involved in the treatment of their spouses, and breast cancer can affect them too. As breast cancer is not a preventable cancer and only women with a high lifetime risk of developing breast cancer can be identified, there is an urgent need to follow region-specific screening protocols; public awareness needs to be increased as well. Ignorance plays a huge role in the neglect and late diagnosis of breast cancer. Many women are hesitant about sharing their health issues. This can only be overcome by education, awareness, and female empowerment. Delay in treatment can result in the progression of the stage of cancer with an associated decrease in survival.

When talking about breast cancer, one needs to be aware of the fact that **'Biology is the KING of the Tumor.'** Biology dictates the course of the disease, treatment outcomes, and longevity in a breast cancer patient. It is wrong to think that biopsy can cause the spread of the disease.

If a patient deteriorates, it may be because of tumor biology.

Nowadays, the use of the internet and social media very often influences our behavior and decision-making, and this is also true when we are sick. Blindly following the internet can be a disadvantage. People tend to forget that doctors have obviously studied the subject. Nobody can vouch for the quality and credibility of the content available online.

While it can provide you with information from credible sources, it can also get you links to some sketchy websites that have bogus information. Seeking treatment with alternative medicine in the place of standard care leads to delayed presentation and ultimately worst outcomes in breast cancer. There are so many pseudo-experts available. So be careful when reading online resources or taking advice from society on breast cancer. King George's Medical University, Lucknow, is a government hospital, and we provide almost free treatment to cancer patients. There is always a huge rush waiting to avail of the investigation and treatment facilities. In many societies, it is considered a stigma to get treatment from a government hospital. Many patients travel from my state to large metro cities like Bangalore, New Delhi, Ahmedabad, and Mumbai.

Two years ago, we started the Lucknow Breast Cancer Support Group (LBCSG). The group comprises survivors, patients, and their primary caregivers, who are here to help and support every patient who has lost hope and is going through a difficult time. The objective of the group is to provide information and support with respect to treatments, coping strategies, and rehabilitation to patients and caregivers. The LBCSG helps to increase the bonding between patients and caregivers, helps patients connect with other cancer survivors, and provides psychological and social support to improve the overall quality of their lives. Our message to the survivors is this: You can lead a 'normal life' after breast cancer! I hope that this book will be a useful information source on breast cancer for everybody and will also be useful in creating awareness. The success stories of survivors will help generate 'Hope' and 'Confidence' in patients suffering from this disease.

ABOUT THE AUTHOR

Dr. Anand Kumar Mishra (MS, MCh, MCh, FACS, FICS) is a specialist endocrine and breast surgeon currently working as Professor and Head of the Department of Endocrine Surgery at the King George's Medical University, Lucknow, Uttar Pradesh, India.

He has been awarded various travel awards by many international organizations for his breast cancer–related work. He is the recipient of the IDEA award by the American Society of Oncology, International Guest Scholarship by the American College of Surgeons, Young Surgeon Travel Grant by the Japan Surgical Society, ICMR Travel Grant, Breast Surgery International Travel Grant, and Developing Nations Fellowship of the European Breast Cancer Conference. He is a very popular teacher and a regular faculty at almost all the national conferences of his specialty. He is the chief editor of Endocrine Surgery – South Asian Perspective, a textbook on Endocrine Surgery published by CRC Press, and A Clinical Guide to Thyroidectomies from Nova Science Publishers, USA, and the co-editor of IAES Textbook of Endocrine Surgery from Jaypee group, New Delhi. He has written chapters for several books, published more than eighty papers in reputed scientific journals, and presented more than a hundred research papers at national and international conferences.

Dr. Anand Mishra founded the 'Lucknow Breast Cancer Support Group', which provides hope, courage, encouragement, and practical support to breast cancer patients and survivors. He is actively involved in breast cancer–related awareness activities and has organized many awareness campaigns.

Dr. Anand Mishra is also keen on athletics and basketball and has won numerous prizes in sports. He was also a member of the Nepal Earthquake Rescue Team from his university in 2015.

www.ingramcontent.com/pod-product-compliance
Lightning Source LLC
Chambersburg PA
CBHW030007290326
41934CB00005B/253